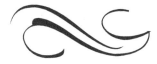

The Dr. Sebi Compendium

• A Healing Journey •

The 3 in 1 Book with Herbs, Cures, Treatments, Diet, Recipes, Detox Plan, and Everything Else you Need to Know about Dr. Sebi Methods and Philosophy

Innovative Wellness

First Printing Edition, 2020
ISBN 978-1-80132-422-9

Printed in the United States of America
Available from Amazon.com and other retail outlets

Table of Contents

INTRODUCTION OF "THE DR. SEBI APPROVED HERBS HANDBOOK"

W e always regard diet as a short, grueling period after which we will find ourselves in perfect shape. But, a good diet is actually a change in lifestyle, that does not only restrict the consumption of harmful food to get in better shape, but to lead a longer, healthier, and stronger life.

That is exactly what the Dr. Sebi Diet offers.

Dr. Sebi, or Alfredo Bowman, the renowned herbalist creator of the diet suffered himself from a host of diseases that made his life unbearable: diabetes, obesity, high blood pressure. He wanted to find a permanent, stable cure to his problems, without relying on medications or on the health care system, that so often has disappointed and abandoned African-Americans.

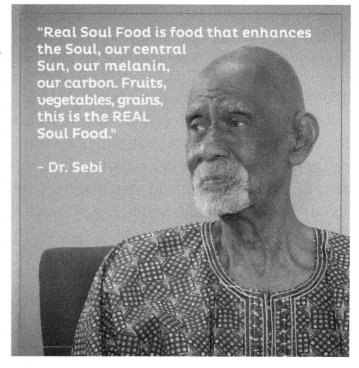

"Real Soul Food is food that enhances the Soul, our central Sun, our melanin, our carbon. Fruits, vegetables, grains, this is the REAL Soul Food."

- Dr. Sebi

Dr. Sebi 's diet focuses on consuming plant-based and avoiding refined foods.

It is simply a vegan, plant-based diet that restricts foods and products made by industrialized processes.

Dr. Sebi posited that you create an alkaline state in your body when you do these two things, which makes it impossible for disease to reside in. All the products and foods on the diet are carefully chosen to minimize acidity in your food and your body mucus.

While he was highly criticized for his diet and ostracized by the scientific community, his claims turned out to be true: refined sugar and carbs are not only completely useless to our nutrition, but also the main cause of diabetes and cardiovascular diseases. A low-carb, whole natural diet is the only permanent, medication-free lifestyle you can adopt to cure these diseases; and the Dr. Sebi's diet is the perfect template for it.

The mucus reduction alkaline diet involves eating from a proprietary nutritional guide and food list, based on 40+ years of research identifying non-hybrid, alkaline foods while also consuming herbal essences of Dr. Sebi cell food.

Dr. Sebi's research showed that the disease is a result of mucus and acidity in the body and argued that in an alkaline environment, diseases could not exist. His plan, which requires a very strict nutritional regime and supplements, promises to detoxify the disease body and restore alkalinity.

The diet restricts any kind of animal products, and overall focuses on vegan eating but with much more stringent rules. It is essentially a raw vegan diet that does not focus on portion control, but rather on eating the right food. It might seem quite restrictive, but as you will find out in the last chapter there are some amazingly tasty recipes on the diet, that will soon make you forget the highly refined, processed food we are used to, and that will help you lead a healthier and better life.

A central part to his health and nutrition plan is also the use of particular herbs, that he carefully chose during his many years of research in the field of herbal traditional medicine. He developed a new methodology and system to repair the human body with herbs.

He personally studied and observed plants and herbs in North America, Central and South America, Africa and the Caribbean, and developed a unique style and methodology for treating the human body with herbs that are rooted in his more than 30 years of empirical experience, knowledge, and experience.

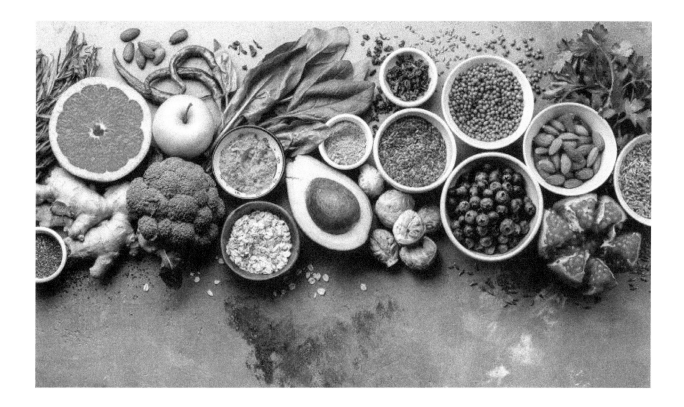

CHAPTER 1

What is Dr. Sebi Diet and How It Works

D r. Sebi felt that the Western solution to illness was unsuccessful. He believed that acidity and mucus — which bred bacteria and viruses — induced sickness.

A big dietary hypothesis is that illness can exist only in acidic conditions. In order to avoid or eliminate the disease, the purpose of the diet is to maintain alkaline conditions in the body. The official website of the diet offers botanical medicines helping to detoxify the body.

The platform does not relate any literature that supports its safety advantage claims. The Commission states that the Food and Drug Administration (FDA) has not studied the statements. The creators understand that they are not professional practitioners and do not intend to provide professional recommendations.

Methodology

Sometimes just one step, can get you to a state you had only dreamed about. Going on an alkaline diet will be the battle that ultimately contributes to a balanced lifestyle. An alkaline diet is an assumption that certain products, such as berries, vegetables, roots, and legumes, leave an alkaline residue or ash behind in the body.

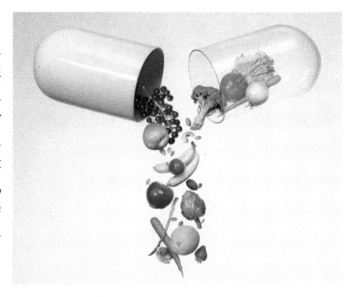

The body is strengthened by the key ingredients of rock, such as calcium, magnesium, titanium, zinc, and copper. To avoid chronic diseases such as asthma, malnutrition, exhaustion, and even cancer, an alkaline diet is the perfect prevention tool.

Here are ten strategies to adopt the alkaline diet effectively.

1. **Drink water** - Water is probably our body's most important (after oxygen) resource. Hydration in the body is vital as the water content determines the body's chemistry. Drink between 8-10 glasses of water to keep the body well hydrated (filtered to cleaned).

2. **Avoid acidic drinks like Tea, coffee, or soda** - Our body also attempts to regulate the acid and alkaline content. There is no need to blink in carbonated drinks as the body refuses carbon dioxide as waste!

3. **Breathe** - Oxygen is the explanation that our body works, and if you provide the body with adequate oxygen, it should perform better. Sit back and enjoy two to five minutes of slow breaths. Nothing is easier than you can perform Yoga.

4. **Avoid food with preservatives and food colors** - Our body has not been programmed to absorb such substances, and the body then absorbs them or retains them as fat, and they do not damage the liver. Chemicals create acids, such that the body neutralizes them either by generating cholesterols or blanching iron from the RBCs (leading to anemia) or by extracting calcium from bones (osteoporosis).

5. **Avoid artificial sweeteners** - These sweeteners, which tend to be high in low fat, are potentially detrimental to the body. In addition, Saccharin, a primary ingredient in sweeteners, triggers cancer. Keep away from these things, therefore. Go for less healthy food, still a decent one.

6. **Exercise-** The alkaline and the acidic element will also be matched. This is not just a question of taking in alkaline milk. A little acid (because of muscles) often regulates natural bodywork.

7. **Satiate your urges for a snack by eating vegetables, or soaked nuts** - Whenever we are thirsty, we still consume a little fast food. Establish a tradition of consuming fresh vegetables or almonds, even walnuts.

8. **Eat the right mix of food** ~ The fats and proteins of carbohydrates need a specific atmosphere when digested. And don't eat it all at once. Evaluate the nutritional composition and balance it accurately to create the best combination of all the nutrients you consume.

9. **Use Green powders as alternates to food** ~ This tends to improve the alkaline quality of the body.

10. **Sleep well** ~ Seek to escape the pain. Our mind regulates the digestive system, and only when in a relaxed, focused condition can you realize it functions properly. Relax, then, and remain safe!

Nutrition Guide

Dr. Sebi's Nutrition Guide includes a variety of guidelines, such as:

- Only eat nourishments recorded in the guide;
- Drink 1 gallon of common spring water day by day;
- Avoid creature items, half and half nourishments, and liquor;
- Avoid utilizing a microwave, which will "slaughter your food;"
- Avoid canned and seedless natural products.

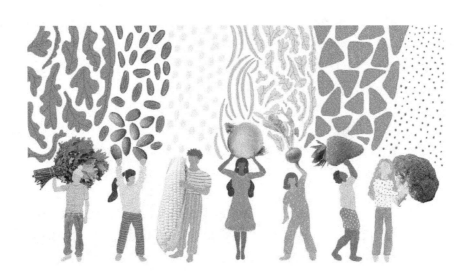

The Doctor Sebi Diet, is it Safe?

Research suggests, however, that a diet focused on plants will improve wellbeing. There are other issues that we will address in the following segment.

Other health benefits of herbal diets can include:

- Loss of weight -in the 2015 report, a vegan diet contributed to greater loss of weight than other, less restricted diets. After six months, participants lost up to 7.5 percent of their body weight on a vegan diet.
- Appetite management — A 2016 analysis of young male participants showed that after consuming a meal containing peas and beans, they feel more relaxed and happier than after a meal containing beef.
- Microbiome modification – the word "microbiome" generally applies to intestinal microorganisms. A research study in 2019 showed that a plant-based diet could favorably modify the microbiome and contribute to lower disease risk. However, more work would be required to validate this.
- Decreased risk of illness — A plant-based diet study in 2017 found that the potential for coronary heart failure may be lowered by 40 percent and the likelihood of developing metabolic syndrome and type 2 diabetes by around half.

Dr. Sebi's lifestyle encourages people to consume natural foods and removes packaged products. A 2017 study showed that a decrease in the consumption of refined foods would increase the overall nutritional consistency of the U.S. diet.

Dr. Sebi's diet is stringent and does not contain adequate significant nutrients that are not explicitly identified on the diet webpage.

If a person follows the diet, he or she may benefit from a healthcare provider who can advise on appropriate supplements.

CHAPTER 2

Alkaline Herbs and Spice

Herbs Self-Cleanse and Revitalize Your Body

Detoxification or cleansings depend on the types of fasting that you desire and trust me, it will do you better if you consume some of the cleansing herbs during your fasting period. However, if you decide to do the water fasting for a week, then throughout that week, you should consume only water and the cleansing herbs in a tea and nothing else should be consume

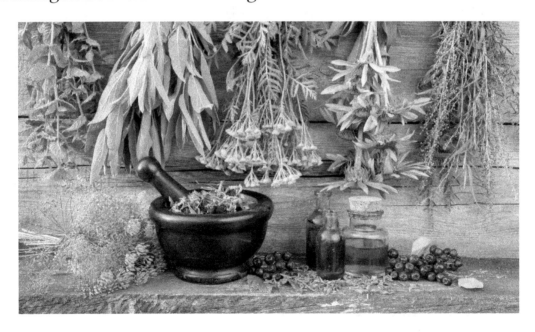

List and Use

1.   **Cascara sagrada** is a shrub plant, that most people only know it as "dietary supplement," and was allowed to be sold in the pharmacies as over the counter drugs. However, in 2002, FDA declares that it doesn't meet the standards to be sold as over the counter drugs (OTC) or prescription drugs. Before then, the dietary supplement or the bark of Cascara Sagrada was used as a purgative for constipation. One sweet thing about this shrub is the fact that it is a bitter less extract that can also be used as a flavoring agent.

2.   **Rhubarb Root** is the root and underground stem (that is, rhizome) of the Rhubarb plant. This plant's root has been used by the traditional Chinese people as a medication for the treatment of digestive tract disorder which include; stomach pain, constipation, menstrual cramps (dysmenorrhea), diarrhea, swelling of pancreas etc. The stems of this plant is also used as a flavoring agent and mostly used to make pie and serves as great recipes. Because of the chemicals that Rhubarb root contains such as fiber, research has it that it a potent laxative has the potency to reduce swelling, treat cold sores and improves the tone and health of the digestive tract, cleans heavy metal and harmful bacteria, improve the general movement of the intestines and also, reduce cholesterol levels.

3.   **Prodigiosa** is also known as 'Brickellia Grandiflora herb' it is a flowering plant/shrub from the daisy family and native to Mexico and California. These plant/shrubs have been use by the Mexican as a tea for the treatment of; diarrhea, diabetes and stomach pain. Research carried on Prodigiosa shows that, the plant is an antioxidant, it contains chemical compound that aid in stimulating the pancreatic gland to secret and reduces or lowers blood sugar level, aid the digestion of fat in the gallbladder and also, improves the healthiness of the stomach digestive system.

4.   **Burdock root** is the root of a plant called Burdock that can be found all over the world. Virtually everything about Burdock is important as its root is used as food and medicine and it leaf, and seed are used for medicinal purpose. A lot of people believe that consuming Burdock orally, helps to increase the flow of urine, eradicate germs, purify blood, prevent and treat cancer, joint pain, cold, diabetes, anorexia, fever, bladder infections, syphilis, stomach and intestinal complaints. This plant does not stop there as it also helps in treating and preventing of skin diseases such as;

acne and psoriasis. Burdock also help in boosting of sex drive (libido), lowering of high blood pressure and cleansing of the liver and lymphatic system.

5.   **Dandelion** is a flowering plant also known as "Taraxacum officinale" it is a native to Europe. It is commonly found in the mild climates of the northern hemisphere. These flowering plants have been in used for centuries before now for the treatment of swelling (inflammation) of the pancreas, cancer, tonsils (tonsillitis), acne, bladder or urethra, digestive and liver disorder. Because of the vitamin (A, B, C, E and K), mineral (iron, potassium, magnesium and calcium) and other compound (Polyphenols, Chicoric and Chlorogenic acid) that Dandelion contains, research has it that it has the potency to detoxify gallbladder, kidney and purifies blood. It also dissolves kidney stones, treat and prevent diabetes and relief liver and urinary disorder. It also contains chemicals that may increase urine production which helps in cleansing the urinary tract and prevent crystals from forming in the urine.

6.   **Elderberry** is also known as European elderberry or black elder or Sambucus nigra. It is a flowering plant that belongs to Adoxaceae family and the native to Europe. These flowering plants are common in Europe and many other parts of the world. This plant can grow as long as 9 meters. That is 30feet tall and has a lot of clusters (white or cream-colored flowers) which is known as elderflowers. The leaves of elderberry have been used for many years for the treatment of pain, inflammation, swelling, and to stimulate urine production and to induce sweat. The bark is not left behind as it was also used as laxative, diuretic, and to induce vomiting.

7.   **Guaco** is a climbing plant that is also known as "Guace or Vedolin or Cepu or Bejuco de finca or Liane Francois or Cipo caatinga and other names. This climbing plant is rich with various minerals and compound. It is from the family of Asteraceae, and species of cordifolia. Its leaf is very medicinal and nutritional.

8.   **Mullein** is a flavorful beverage plant that is also known as 'Aaron's rod, Candlewick, American mullein, Adam's flannel, Denseflower mullein, Candleflower, European or orange mullein etc. this flavorful beverage plant has been used for centuries before now for the treatment of diverse sicknesses, which include; asthma, tuberculosis, pneumonia, chills flu, gastrointestinal bleeding, colds, chronic coughs and others.

Natural Herbal Tea

According to Dr. Sebi, it is important to maintain a "consistent use of natural botanical remedies' and doing so will cleanse and detoxify the body.

While using herbs and natural remedies is an important step in your journey to greater health, you must also remember to make the right adjustments to your eating habits by following the recommended foods list.

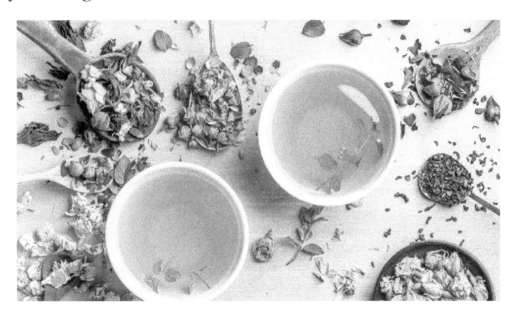

List and Use

We have seen that a plant-based nutrition is fundamental for a healthy diet. But when we talk about plants, we can't consider only fruits and vegetables, in fact there is also an incredible variety of herbs with a powerful alkaline effect. We need to understand how important they could be for our health: they have a real healing effect that prevents and revers many diseases.

Herbal medicine is a very ancient practice and it consist in a series of healing techniques based on plants; also, the official modern medicine is aware of the extraordinary properties of many plants and it uses them for many common drugs.

We can assume most of their macronutrients in a totally natural way simply through infusions, so we can't neglect them in our alkaline diet. I want to mention a very famous plant: chamomile. Many people use it to relax or sleep, but very few people know its important alkaline effect: when you're stressed or worried, your body increases the production of acid, so a chamomile tea, thanks to its relaxing effect, helps your body to balance its pH value. Moreover, chamomile fights arachidonic acid and the result is an important anti-inflammatory effect.

Alfalfa, also called Lucerne, is a less know herb with an incredible high level of nutrients. Its name means "Father of All Foods", in fact it contains a wide variety of vitamins, minerals, protein and essential amino acids. Beyond its alkalizing effect, it allows you to reset your metabolism and stay away from different common diseases. More in details, it can:

- lower the cholesterol level

- increase immune system functionality

- clean the blood

- support digestion

- alleviate allergies

- relieve all forms of arthritis

- relieve headaches and migraines

You should drink alfalfa tea daily, mixing it with another flavored tea if you prefer, since alfalfa is very mild in flavor. Or you could take this herb in capsule form. Whatever you decide, remember that this herb should never be missing, it is one of the biggest secrets for an incredible healthy life!

Dandelion is another alkaline herb that you can eat as a tea or also as a salad. It is an effective aid against kidney stones, it promotes weight loss and it contains potent Antioxidants. Dandelion is very rich in vitamin C and folic acid, which are susceptible to heat: for this reason, I suggest you consume this herb as a fresh vegetable, preparing delicious salads with other vegetables. Dandelion is of course very cheap, you can easily collect it in the fields or cultivate it in your garden, so you should seriously consider adding this herb in your daily healthy diet.

A particular and almost unknown medicinal herb tea is the one based on red clover. It contains isoflavones, natural phytoestrogens with high antioxidant effects, used for cancer prevention, indigestion, asthma and bronchitis. Red clover is particularly suitable for women, because it promotes female reproductive health and it may reduce risk of breast cancer.

There are many herbs that are totally undervalued: usually people think that their only purpose is to add flavor to our dishes, but they add much more than that. I think for example of parsley, basil, cilantro, oregano, sage and thyme.

Nobody knows that parsley contains more vitamin C than oranges! Similarly, it has a very high percentage of vitamin K and a lot of iron.

Basil releases into our body high quantities of eugenol, a powerful anti-inflammatory, while oregano is one of the best sources of the free-radical fighters.

Among the other alkaline herbs, that we can use to prepare excellent infusions, we can mention lime, sarsaparilla, verbena, sage, and laurel.

Laurel is a valid ally against respiratory diseases like flu, bronchitis, cough and pharyngitis. Moreover, it has positive effects for the treatment of vascular problems and arteriosclerosis. You should consider also to buy the essential oil, which has antibacterial and antitussive properties.

10~Day Detox Plans with Herbs

Day	Morning	Evening
1	Savory	Bird Pepper of Africa
2	Thyme & Dill	Fresh Cayenne
3	Bay Leaves	Sage
4	Sweet Basil & Basil	Achiote
5	Tarragon	Pulverized Onion
6	Cloves	Habanero
7	Oregano	Sweet Sensational Savor
8	Pulverized Granulated Seaweed	Purified Cactus Agave Syrup
9	Purified Sea Salt	Date Sugar
10	Kelp	Nori

CHAPTER 4CHAPTER 4

How to Follow The Diet

Rules to Follow

To follow Dr. Sebi's diet, you need to strictly adhere to his rules, which are present on his website. Here is a list of his guidelines below:

1. Do not eat or drink any product or ingredient not mentioned in the approved list for the diet. It is not recommended and should never be consumed when following the diet.

2. You have to drink almost one gallon (or more than three liters) of water every day. It is recommended to drink spring water.

3. You have to take Dr. Sebi's mixtures or products one hour before consuming your medications.

4. You can take any of Dr. Sebi's mixtures/products together without any worry.

5. You need to follow the nutritional guidelines stringently and punctually take Dr. Sebi's mixtures/products daily.

6. You are not allowed to consume any animal-based food or hybrid products.

7. You are not allowed to consume alcohol or any kind of dairy product.

8. You are not allowed to consume wheat, only natural growing grains as listed in the nutritional guide

9. The grains mentioned in the nutritional guide can be available in different forms, like pasta and bread, in different health food stores. You can consume them.

10. Do not use fruits from cans; also, seedless fruits are not recommended for consumption.

11. You are not allowed to use a microwave to reheat your meals.

How Prepare the Body

It should be clear that it is a restrictive diet low in calories. Many people believe that because of this reason, it cannot be used as a standard way to lose weight as it puts too much stress on the body of a new dieter. Because it is low in calories and an intensive diet, weight loss can be seen, but the person needs to assess whether they are capable of handling a low caloric diet. Being too ambitious with this diet might turn fatal, so if you want to try the diet, be careful!

This diet has been suggested to be followed throughout one's entire life, which might not be possible for a new dieter. With any diet, if you start cutting foods strongly and then revert to your old routine of eating unhealthy meals, the chances are that the weight loss and benefits you see will get reversed. This is a risk in this diet as well. When starting, set reasonable goals and don't go too strongly. Let your body first get used to it and then start setting up more ambitious goals.

Meal Plan

Starting the diet can be daunting, so here is a list of meal ideas that you can copy from. For the first few days, follow it so that you get used to the diet.

Breakfast

1. Banana pancakes with agave syrup (more than one is recommended).

2. A strawberry and banana smoothie with added hemp seeds and water.

3. Cooked quinoa with coconut milk (pure) and agave syrup for sweetness (add a fruit of your choice as well).

Lunch

1. A salad made up of kale, tomatoes, onions, avocados, and chickpeas with olive oil and dressing of herbs.

2. A pizza made with spelt flour, Brazil nut cheese topped with different vegetables like tomatoes, etc.

3. A pasta made of spelt with different vegetables, and lime and olive oil dressings.

Evening Snack

1. A smoothie made by cucumbers, kale, a few pieces of ginger, and one or two apples.

2. Herbal tea accompanied by the fruit of your choice.

3. Blueberry muffins made by spelt and teff flour, coconut milk (pure), agave syrup, and blueberries.

Dinner

1. A wild rice stir-fry with vegetables of your choice.

2. A burger made up of spelt flour bread; tomatoes, onions, and kale as vegetables; and a chickpea patty.

3. Thick vegetable soup made up of zucchini, mushrooms, peppers, spices, sea salt, onions, and seaweed powder.

Drink Water

Smoothies are a drink, and by drinking them, you are ultimately fulfilling your water intake for the day. Dr. Sebi's diet requires you to drink one gallon of water daily, but that can be difficult. Dehydration is a serious problem that can lead to anxiety. To prevent that, you need to drink lots of water, which the smoothie diet helps you with.

What You Should Not Eat

Foods that are not listed in the nutritional guide are not allowed to be consumed. Some examples of such foods are given below:

1. Any canned product, be it fruits or vegetables, listed in the nutritional guide

2. Seedless fruits like grapes

3. Eggs are not permitted

4. Any type of dairy product is not allowed

5. Fish is not permitted

6. Any type of poultry is not to be eaten

7. Red meat is strictly banned

8. Soy products, which are a replacement for meat, are also banned

9. Processed foods are not allowed

10. Restaurant foods and delivered foods are not to be consumed

11. Hybrid and fortified foods are not permitted

12. Wheat is not permitted

13. White sugar is strictly banned

14. Alcohol is banned

15. Yeast and its products are not allowed

16. Baking powder is not permitted

Some other foods and ingredients have been cut off. You only need to follow the nutritional guide to know what you have to eat.

Alkaline Meal Plan

Among the diverse body parts, the liver is among one of the significant organs, for it has considerable capacity in body detoxification. Through this body detoxification, synthetics and other outside substances like poisons and even defecation, pee, and sweat are expelled from the body. These substances originate from the unsafe nourishments that we eat like handled and non-regular rich nourishments, liquor drinks that we devour, cigarettes that we smoke, and even drugs that we expend for anti-infection treatment and hormone elective drugs. These substances are the ones that our bodies attempt to take out every day.

When there are many harming materials inside the body, the liver needs to keep keeping up until its ability runs out. When this is dismissed, vast amounts of poisons can be gathered in the body and will cause many body issues and diseases. To anticipate this and keep up excellent health, we should experience a detoxification diet and take significant consideration of our liver.

A liver detoxification plan can be completed either on a three-day, seven-day, or twenty-one-day program. This depends on a firm focus on a diet with unprocessed and natural foods grown from the ground, entire grains, and water cure with enough measure of water or liquid other option. Nourishments that are wealthy in fat or sugar, caffeine, liquor drinks, unnatural and human-made nourishment, drugs, and low-quality nourishments would all be able to must be put to a stop, at any rate, seven days before the diet plan.

One to Three Days: This is the period to start your fluid diet plan where you need to drink around ten to twelve glasses of water ordinarily alongside frequently crushed lime juice. Even though it can indeed be challenging to execute this diet because of the weariness and slightness, light exercise can be included as a request to affix the method of flushing the poisons out of the body. Additionally, you should shun taking in any sort of milk or dairy item.

Four to Six Days: Fresh organic products, vegetables, and entire grains can be expended like celery, apples, carrots, oranges, which would all be able to be blended into one juice. The juice can incorporate your selection of leafy foods. Even though healthy nourishments are devoured, there are as yet liquid choices, for example, natural teas for around a few cups every day. Concerning suppers, they can incorporate cut and bubbled vegetables like celery, carrots, broccoli, and spinach. Besides, you can likewise utilize soups that can be taken in at regular intervals.

Seven days: Along with the leafy foods, the liquids are expended together. They would all be able to be arranged by having them crude or steamed. Additionally, you can consume rosemary tea and dandelion options, which can be useful for this period.

You can generally change the sorts of foods grown from the ground that you will use as long as you oblige the strategy. When the seventh day is a doe, you can participate in the typical diet; finally, however, there is still a restriction on liquor consumption for around one entire week after the detoxification diet. You have to end the food once you feel torment, disorder, and squeamishness. Most likely, this detoxification diet can have an enormous impact on the advancement and support of a healthy lifestyle.

Instructions to Detox Your Body with Alternative Therapies

Conventional Chinese Medicine (TCM) is a fantastic asset when figuring out how to detox your body, and is mainly prescribed for treating stomach related issue, for example, bad-tempered inside syndrome; ceaseless skin conditions like dermatitis; weariness and despair; hormonal awkward nature, for example, PMS; endometriosis and poor sperm tally, and barrenness (both male and female). It can create results with interminable conditions that Western methods neglect to help. At the point when joined with a detox diet, it can make perceptible upgrades to a people's health and prosperity.

Self-finding and treatment of ailments are not suggested; however, at some TCM focuses, you can portray your side effects to the specialist behind the counter and get a suitable cure on the spot. TCM can be useful for treating individuals experiencing withdrawal from drug and liquor addictions. Liquor makes liver and nerve bladder uneven characters, which realizes a mix of unnecessary moistness and warmth.

Numerous drugs are prepared through the liver, making it warmed and blocked, so the liver's blood gets frail and insufficient. TCM equations center on clearing and supporting the liver and nerve bladder, while simultaneously treating the heart, to help quiet the brain and sensory system. Consolidating TCM with figuring out how to detox your body yourself is probably the best thing you can accomplish for your health.

CHAPTER 5

Advantages of the Dr. Sebi Alkaline

The alkaline diet has a lot of benefits in maintaining a person's health. Its benefits are mostly provided by decreasing the consumption of unhealthy foods and eating more vegetables and fruits. To get the most out of any diet regimen is to accompany it with other healthy routines like exercise. It is a great idea to start an alkaline diet to improve your everyday life as we are drowning in bad health with our lazy lifestyle and fast foods. The following is a list of benefits that can be provided by this diet.

Weight loss

This diet was not made with weight loss in mind, but because it is extremely restrictive, you will see weight loss. Also, one of the main reasons that this diet is effective in reducing weight is that it makes people stop consuming Western foods, which are highly caloric, oily, and sugary.

Weight loss occurs when you eat less or equal amounts of calories that you can burn. If you follow this diet—which is low in sugar, fat, and processed foods—you can get your perfect body.

Any diet whose main component is eating unprocessed plant-based foods is shown to reduce the causes of heart disease and also obesity.

The foods listed in this diet are low in calories, except for some nuts and oils. Even if you eat a large quantity of them due to excessive hunger, they will not overthrow your daily calorie intake by much. If you eat other types of food, they will result in weight gain and excessive eating.

A constant state of weight loss can only be possible if you plan your servings and portion out ingredients properly. The diet does not provide this information, so it will depend on your management skills to plan your meals.

Improves kidney function

Acidic diets mostly affect the health of the kidneys and damages the layers inside the organ system. To promote kidney health, the pH of the urine mustn't be acidic. By consuming a lot of alkaline food and removing acidic foods from our daily routine, we can reach this pH in which our kidneys remain safe and healthy. Alkaline diets do not affect the pH of the blood, but it can significantly affect the urine. Drinking a lot of water alongside this diet can improve kidneys even more.

If you're suffering from any chronic kidney disease, then you should know that this diet is not targeted for you. You can follow the diet after consulting your doctor first.

Reduces the risk of cancer

There are almost no significant studies that show that an alkaline diet leads to decreased cases of cancer. However, there have been lessons that show that if a person were to eat less meat and increase their consumption of fresh fruits and vegetables, then that person is at a lower risk of cancer.

Also, another study showed that having more vitamins, like vitamin C, in your diet can prevent cancer. Generally, eating more fruits and vegetables and consuming less high fatty and sugary foods leads to a reduction in developing cancer.

Reduces the risk of heart disease

Heart disease is the major cause of death in the world. It is mainly caused by eating lots of fat and oily foods, which results in the development of plaque and blockage of arteries. In this diet, the consumption of fats goes down significantly, decreasing the chances of developing heart disease.

It has also been shown that growth hormones are related to decreased rates of heart disease. An alkaline diet increases the levels of growth hormones, so, in turn, it decreases heart disease as well.

Reduces the risk of muscle degradation

When we grow old or stop using our muscles, we tend to increase muscle loss. However, there was a study conducted in 2013 showing that people who follow the alkaline diet could decrease muscle degradation. The diet is low in red meat, so there is a risk of decreasing muscle mass and strength.

People eat more fruits and vegetables

Nowadays, people lean towards the fast and tasty treats and forget about eating fresh produce. Following this diet will lead to people consuming their daily requirement of vegetables and fruits. With the increase in their intake, we take in all their benefits and nutrition as well.

Increases intestinal health

With the addition of whole grains, there is a list of nuts and seeds that you can eat on this diet. It contributes to an increase in fiber intake, which increases the health of small and large intestines. It helps manage regular bowel movements, which reduces the risk of developing many diseases.

Decreases the harmful effects of processed foods

Processed foods have been linked to increased sugar intake and fat content. They also contain lots of calories but have very low nutritional value. Many additives and preservatives that have no purpose in our body are eliminated from our diets if we strictly avoid processed foods.

It helps the brain

The growth hormone is not only related to a better heart condition but also helps manage the health of the mind. It is related to an increase in memory and cognition. Eating a healthy diet rich in fruits and vegetables leads to better brain functioning.

It may improve back pain

Alkaline minerals are related to the reduction of back pain, but whether alkaline foods provide the same results has yet to be determined. There is a decent chance that the diet has similar effects.

Decreases the level of inflammation

Diets rich in fresh fruits and vegetables show a great decrease in oxidative stress and inflammation. This leads to less discomfort and fewer diseases developing in our bodies.

CHAPTER 6

Tips for starting the Dr. Sebi Diet

D r. Sebi's nutritional guide is quite strict, so one has to be mentally and emotionally prepared before starting this diet. It sounds impossible to follow, but once you get all the information you need, you will find yourself set for the journey.

The critical aspect of eating is eating correctly. 3-5 meals a day, chewing well, and not drinking water before your meals are the universal rules to follow, on a diet or not!

Digestion

Humans need food to live. The food we can find in nature: fruits, vegetables, fish, and other animals.

Digestion is a form of catabolism that helps us breakdown large food molecules into small soluble molecules that will be absorbed through the small intestines into the bloodstream and then into the cells, tissues, and organs.

The digestive system starts with chewing. The contact of food with the saliva starts the digestion and provides the ideal conditions of pH. The food transfers to the stomach, where, with the aid of gastric acids and enzymes, is transformed into smaller molecules.

After a few hours, the resulting liquid enters the duodenum, where, with the assistance from pancreatic digestive enzymes and bile juice from the liver, it continues to be digested. Once digestion is over, the nutrients are absorbed into the blood.

So, proteins are converted to amino acids, glucides to glucose, and lipids to fatty acids.

Metabolism

The metabolism is a set of chemical reactions in any organism. It helps us:

- converse the essential nutrients from foods into energy

- converse foods into proteins, nucleic acids, lipids, and carbohydrates

- eliminate the nitrogenous waste

Each human needs food to live, have the power to work, fight harmful elements, revitalize cells and tissues, and eliminate toxins from the body.

Finding food was always a problem for humans. The first people on Earth only used a vegetarian regimen. In time, they started hunting and fishing. When they discovered fire, people began to vary their diet- now they had tools to grow crops and raise animals.

In the 19th century, people started to use refined products such as sugar, flour, and other food concentrates.

In the 20th century, people started to use hybrid and genetically modified foods due to selective breeding and mutation breeding.

Why is food so important?

We need food to obtain the lipids, proteins, vitamins, minerals, and carbohydrates our body needs daily to synthesize into nutrients.

With the help of digestion, we can obtain the essential enzymes, amino acids, and other nutrients vital for our body's functioning. They will keep us healthy and robust.

With the help of metabolism, we make the most of the nutrients. In small words, the faster our cells, tissues, and organs synthesize the small molecules, the more our body stays in shape. There will be no time for BAT (brown adipose tissue) to form.

Mindset

Plants are probably the best choice for our nutrition. Dr. Sebi certainly thought so. In my humble opinion, he was entirely right.

Natural foods can only help us. Processed foods are full of additives, salt, sugar, and food preservatives, which are not entirely healthy and maybe a significant aspect of the high level of obesity and other health problems in the US. In the entire world, actually!

One could say: it depends on natural food! Yes, the nutritional guide for Dr. Sebi Diet is restrictive, some ingredients are not that easy to find in any supermarket, but with a bit of patience, you will come to realize that it is not that hard. Mindset is essential, as in anything worth fighting for!

When you want to lose weight, you must consider that restriction is a must, and obstacles will always pop up when least expected.

Try to focus on your goal and not on how limited your meal options are.

Being emotionally ready is a big step ahead. Changing your eating habits is not easy. Daily habits are firmly inserted into our subconscious, so we must take the time to adjust them. Begin with small steps and keep telling yourself that this is the right way to achieve your goals, weight loss, and overall health.

Get support from your family and friends, surround yourself with positive people, and proceed step-by-step. Small changes each day will lead to lifetime healthy eating habits.

Drink more water

We all know how liquids are essential for the proper functioning of our body. The body contains from 55% to 78 % water, depending on body size and age.

We can live with no food for a month, but we don't last more than a few days without water.

Apart from this essential role in life, we use water also to cleanse our bodies. It plays a significant role in maintaining our brain healthy, ensuring proper body functioning, and eliminating toxins from our body.

Keeping well hydrated is vital. Indeed, Dr. Sebi's supplements contain herbs that promote urination to remove toxins, so you must drink more water to replenish the water eliminated.

He advises drinking up to one gallon of water a day. In his opinion, spring water is the best choice since it's naturally alkaline. The tap water can contain high levels of chloride and other contaminants.

Start reading food labels

In any diet that we may follow, knowing what we eat is a must. We will have to deprive ourselves of favorite foods or drinks so that the journey will become tricky.

Starting to read labels will help us understand that junk food is not necessary. It will become easier to let go of some usual foods or snacks which don't contain our needed nutrients.

Knowing what you eat and drink will make you aware of the right food choices you are doing. Changing eating habits will come naturally.

In case of relapse (it's normal to experience it at some point!), the good thing is that you will be completely aware of what you did wrong, what you ate, and shouldn't have.

It may sound stupid, but it's an incentive to change your eating habits for good!

Whole foods

Fresh fruits or vegetables, anything that you like from Dr. Sebi's nutritional guide, of course, are easy to cook, mainly because most of them are best to be consumed raw.

The idea is to avoid packaged or processed foods and slowly introduce into our diet whole foods. Cooking your meals may help you better realize the importance of the diet. Sometimes, you can get great satisfaction from cooking new recipes.

Cooking your meals will make it easier for you to get in control over the foods to eat, so you reclaim your health while trying new approaches to your favorite dishes. The approved ingredients on Dr. Sebi's nutritional guide could add spice to your life.

Snacks

Old habits dye hard! Food is the comfort blanket of the brain. When on a diet, our brain sends us signals of danger, so we "have" to eat in those moments.

Snacking is not necessarily a bad habit. If we have at least 6~7 fruits or vegetable snacks a day, it will work just fine.

Instead of going for a bag of chips, one should eat an apple, some olives, dried fruits, or cherry tomatoes. Our brain is satisfied, our body no longer feels hungry, and we stay fit and slim.

CHAPTER 7

Benefits of Dr. Sebi's Diet

D r. Sebi's Diet is not just another fad. It has numerous benefits besides weight loss. Let's find out how following this vegan, alkaline-based approach to food will completely change our lives.

Weight

Weight loss is the main goal for most of us. Even if Dr. Sebi did not develop this diet for weight loss, we realize that we can lose weight by following his rules.

The diet is based on consuming vegetables and fruits, which are high in vitamins, minerals, fiber, and other compounds associated with reduced inflammation, oxidative stress, and protection against many diseases.

A study has shown that those who ate seven or more servings of fruits and vegetables a day had a lower incidence of cancer and heart disease.

This diet is based on principles opposite to the Western diet since it restricts us from processed foods, dense fats, sugar, salt, and other harmful ingredients.

Detox

The Dr. Sebi Diet is also suitable for eliminating toxins and processed elements from the body.

Our body needs food, and we find all the food we need in nature. But some elements of the foods we eat are harmful. Once they are processed, some become toxic for our bodies. Consuming meats, some vegetables, dairy products, processed foods, and others leads to release of certain harmful elements. These are only a shortcut to chronic diseases.

The purpose of the Dr. Sebi Diet is to eliminate toxins bound to increase the risk of developing such diseases. It will also help us improve our health, vitality, and strength.

Intra-cellular cleansing is necessary to cleanse the body's systems on a cellular level to correct any damage or imbalances. Imbalances refer mainly to nutritional deficiencies and damages to your natural biological structure due to excess toxins, acids, calcification, and mucus build up in your body's systems.

Good eating habits

When one is on a diet, he has to face restriction, straining physical exercises, and, most importantly, dealing with new eating habits.

That is the worst part- getting used to something new, something that "we have to do". When someone tells you to do or not to do something, it may become tricky!

Trust me, I know. The positive aspect is that your body will get used to the new dietary regime in only a few days. Why?

We are vegetarians, even if nobody tells you that. Mother Nature has a way to provide us with all we need. She takes care of plants, animals, and humans. For Amerindians, it represents the goddess of fertility who presides over planting and harvesting.

If nature didn't make it, don't take it!

Anyway, changing your eating habits is not easy, but you will find that it is quite easy if you follow some simple rules for some days. From there on, it will go naturally!

Lower risk of chronic diseases

A potential benefit of this diet is a lower risk of cancer, high blood pressure, heart diseases, and type-2 diabetes. Why? All due to natural foods that contain no harmful nutrients.

CHAPTER 8

Some Disease and Dr Sebi Herbal Cure

Some of the chronic diseases we can cure with Dr. Sebi's diet are:
Hypertension/ High blood pressure.
Hypertension is a long-term health condition in which blood pressure is persistently elevated. It is a significant risk factor for strokes, heart failure, vision loss, and even dementia.

For the cure, we must keep away from meat and alcohol, drink not too much tea, and eat fruits and vegetables approved by Dr. Sebi. The vegetables to eat are olives, wild rice, lettuce, cucumber, bell peppers, kale, squash, valerian, and chickpeas. Dry fruits are the best choice for our diet.

Type-2 diabetes

Type-2 diabetes is a chronic disease that occurs as a result of obesity, especially in people over the age of 40. It is characterized by a lack of insulin, which is a crucial factor for digestion.

To cure diabetes, we must stay away from fried foods, teas with sugar, rice, and lens. The vegetables to eat are kale, cucumber, lettuce, cherry and plum tomatoes, chickpeas, bell peppers, squash, mushrooms, dandelion, and onions.

We can only eat fruits like red raspberry, plums, apples, and seeded key limes.

Sour soups are highly indicated for the cure of type-2 diabetes.

Obesity

Obesity is a chronic ailment in which excess body fat accumulated leads to various conditions, such as type-2 diabetes, cardiovascular diseases, obstructive sleep apnea, osteoarthritis, depression, and even some types of cancer.

It is caused by bad eating habits, inactive lifestyle, genetics, gut flora, mental illnesses, and social determinants.

The best cure for obesity is eating fruits and vegetables, keeping away from meat and alcohol, and drinking plenty of liquids.

Stress ulcer

An ulcer is a discontinuity in the body membrane, which hinders the normal function of the affected organ. Stress ulcer is the most common type of ulcer encountered in all countries.

It affects mainly the stomach and may lead to ulcerative perigastritis, stenosis, and massive bleeding.

Dr. Sebi's cure includes eating vegetables like tomatoes and squash, ripe fruits (apples, peaches, raisins), sour soups, and plenty of herbal teas, especially fennel and chamomile, for their soothing effect.

Constipation

Constipation is a disorder that profoundly affects our well-being. Abdominal pain, bloating, and infrequent bowel movements may lead to other complications, such as hemorrhoids and anal fissure.

Dr. Sebi's cure consists of eating fruits (mainly apples, peaches, plums, figs), vegetables (squash, kale, and chickpeas), basil, nuts, and plenty of herbal teas, especially fennel, dandelion, and chamomile.

Atherosclerosis

Atherosclerosis is a disease in which the arteries narrow, and that may lead to strokes, coronary artery disease, and kidney problems.

Smoking and consumption of alcohol are forbidden. Coffee should be limited, but lettuce tea is a valid help.

In addition to physical exercise, we should eat wild rice, fruits, and vegetables.

Herpes and STDs

Herpes and all STDs are viral infections that can not be defeated by the immune system.

The only means of prevention is safe sex. Dr. Sebi's cure includes herbal teas such as burdock and dandelion, eating a lot of dates, and lettuce.

Gout

Gout is inflammatory arthritis characterized by recurrent intense pain, red, hot, and swollen joints, due to low uric acid levels in the blood. It may lead to kidney disease.

In this case, we should combine fiber with the uric acid in the digestive tract, so it does not form crystals deposits anymore.

The most reliable way to prevent gout is to lose weight, consume lots of vitamins, and avoid alcohol.

According to specialists, dietary supplements do not have any effect on gout, but Dr. Sebi advises us to drink burdock, dandelion, and elderberry teas. Eating alkaline fruits and vegetables also helps to lower the uric acid levels.

GERD (gastroesophageal reflux disease)

GERD is a long-term ailment in which stomach contents rise in the esophagus. The leading cause is inadequate closure of the esophageal sphincter, but obesity, obstructive sleep apnea, and gallstones are also involved.

We must change our lifestyle, eat healthily, start exercising, stop smoking, and most certainly let go of acidic foods. That's why Dr. Sebi's nutritional guide will give us a hand to defeat this ailment.

Asthma

Asthma is a chronic inflammation of the longs, due to excess mucus accumulation, environmental and genetic causes.

It's quite hard to prevent it, but easier to cure. Traditional medicine uses vitamins, fatty acids, respiratory maneuvers, and breathing techniques to maintain the lungs' proper function.

Dr. Sebi advises us to use fennel, anise, chamomile teas, and alkaline fruits and vegetables.

Dr. Sebi's Alkaline Diet: Usefulness and Result

What Is the Result of the Diet?

The human body has a range of pH in which it gives optimum performance. It is slightly alkaline, with a range of 7.25–7.35. Many alkaline diets like this one promise to help the body maintain these slightly alkaline levels. In reality, it does almost nothing to the pH levels of the blood because the body has a built-in process to keep it under control. Regardless, following an alkaline diet leads to many health benefits as it encourages the consumption of fruits and vegetables, unprocessed fresh products, and discourages the use of alcohol and other potentially harmful substances. It also makes you drink lots of water.

This diet results in steady weight loss, decreases the risks of many diseases, and lowers the chances of developing them. Kidney stones and kidney diseases are less frequent. Bones and muscles get stronger. It results in higher functioning of the heart and brain, also lowering the chances of their deterioration. You are less likely to develop type 2 diabetes as it is related to obesity, and this diet helps remove obesity by effective weight loss.

People who believe in Dr. Sebi's diet say that it reduces the built-up acidity in our body. If we stop eating alkaline foods, the acid will start to accumulate, and our body will attract many types of diseases. Eating a constant influx of alkaline foods helps to reduce diseases and acidity.

Who Could Benefit from this Diet?

Almost anyone looking to better their life can follow this diet. Unhealthy eating has become prominent all over the world. People of all ages prefer to practically run away from vegetables and fruits these days. Apart from some popular ingredients, people don't know about the large variety of foods that are available at their disposal. Because of laziness and ignorance, people choose not to look at all of the options that might greatly benefit them and settle for the easiest thing they can get on the plate. Dieting, especially alkaline dieting, which is mainly focused on vegetables and fruits, is a crucial step in improving people's health.

More people are obese than ever before. Heart disease and diabetes are the major causes of death. All these aspects are related to bad eating and can be improved if we switch to a healthy and nutritious eating routine, just like this diet.

The people that can benefit the most are obese people looking for a way to shed some pounds so that they don't invite diseases into their bodies. The diet effectively makes a person lose weight and reach their weight goals, so obese and overweight people can improve their lives significantly. Also, it can help people suffering from heart disease and diabetes. Still, before patients should opt for the diet, it is advised that they seek the guidance of a health professional before adopting such a restrictive and low caloric diet.

Reviews About the Diet

Many people have tried and commented on their diet. The people who started the diet were mostly people looking for an effective weight-loss method. The dieting plan ranges for about four weeks for some people with probably a cheat day or two. A complete strict adaptation of the diet for your whole life, just as you are starting, is a near-impossible thing to do even if you have high motivation.

People switching to the diet for the first time—whose meals consist of meat, rice, and bread, with occasional snacking—found the diet to be very difficult during the first week. Their daily routine was affected as they felt a loss in energy, and they sensed weakness for the first few days. Dieters who took supplements and planned their meals to be rich in calories found that they gained some of their energy back, but it was still not enough. After weeks three and four, the diet became easier to follow. In the end, dieters on average saw a great reduction in their weight— approximately two to four pounds per day, after five or six weeks of dieting was completed.

For most people, shopping for the ingredients was quite expensive. You have to buy whole grain, vegetables, fruits, and also supplements that don't make it financially sustainable. It is already a restrictive diet, which makes the dieter lose motivation even further.

There was a concern about malnutrition among dieters. Because this diet cuts off all sources of protein and other compounds like Vitamin B12, they had to take additional supplements.

CHAPTER 10

Top 10 Foods that Seem Healthy but

You Must Avoid

- **Fruit juice**

Many people start their day with a glass of orange juice. Well, they shouldn't. It takes four oranges to produce a single glass of juice. Although juice is a healthy beverage, unfortunately, all the fiber from the fruit has been discarded. Besides, fruit juice contains almost as much sugar as soft drinks. A better way to start a day would be to eat an orange, not drink a glass of orange juice. That way, you'll get all the vitamins, plus the fiber, and the amount of fructose your liver has to deal with would be minimal.

- **Farmed salmon (Atlantic salmon)**

Most people eat salmon because it's high in omega-3 fatty acids. However, farmed salmon available today have considerably lower levels of these healthy fats than the salmon we could buy only five years ago. The most likely reason for this is that salmon is now fed much less nutritious food. Besides, dioxin levels are ten times higher in farmed salmon than in wild salmon. This is bad news because this chemical is linked to cancer, organ damage, and immune system dysfunction.

- **Artificial sweeteners**

Artificial sweeteners are found in many sugar-free products, et chewing gums, baked goods, jams, etc. They are also what sugar replacements are based on, eg sorbitol, xylitol, mannitol, erythritol, maltitol, lactitol and isomalt. Although these artificial sweeteners are marketed as natural, they are actually heavily processed and are many times produced from GMO ingredients. Long-term use of artificial sweeteners can create an imbalance in your gut flora and contribute to the development of diabetes, gastrointestinal problems, weight gain, etc. On top of that, farmed salmon is regularly treated with banned pesticides. To make things even worse, it recently became legal to produce and sell genetically engineered salmon without having to label it as such.

- **Shrimp**

Farmed shrimps contain a certain food additive that is used to improve the color of shrimp. This additive has estrogen-like effects that can affect the sperm count in men and increase the risk of breast cancer in women. Besides, ponds where shrimps are raised, are often treated with neurotoxic pesticides known to cause certain neurological problems, attention deficit symptoms, impaired memory, etc.

- **Fat-free and low-fat milk**

When raw milk is pasteurized, it loses a lot of its nutrients. Long-life milk is particularly unhealthy because it first has to be dried at temperatures of about 1000 degrees Centigrade, after which water is added to it. Needless to say, no enzymes or any other nutrients can survive these high temperatures.

People usually choose low-fat or fat-free dairy products because they don't want to gain weight. However, what they don't realize is that when fat is removed, carbs or sugar are added. This is done so that milk would have flavor, otherwise, it would taste like water. So, fat-free and low-fat milk contains added sugar, which, if you drink a lot of milk, puts you at risk of developing diabetes or heart disease.

- **Coffee with added flavors**

Black coffee has a number of health benefits and can even protect you from certain liver diseases. However, after sugar, whipped cream or powdered milk has been added to it, it becomes a very unhealthy beverage.

It gets even more unhealthy if you add non-dairy liquid creamers based on corn syrup. Black coffee is the healthiest option because although these additives improve the taste of coffee, they also contribute to increased liver fat and some gastrointestinal problems.

- **Seitan**

We usually think of seitan as a healthy alternative to meat protein. However, it is simply wheat gluten. This means that even if you are not allergic to gluten but you often eat seitan, you may develop gluten intolerance symptoms. Besides, seitan contains a lot of sodium, over 500 milligrams per 100 grams.

- **Canned green beans**

For some reason, U.S.-grown canned green beans are some of the most toxic canned foods there are. This food is treated with some of the most dangerous pesticides and eating just one serving a day, puts you at risk of developing cancer and having other health problems. Besides, all cans are lined with materials that contain Bisphenol A. This is a synthetic estrogen that can create fertility problems for both men and women. Unless you can find fresh or frozen green beans, this is one of the foods you must avoid at all costs.

- **Diet soda**

The main reason you should avoid diet soda is that it's full of artificial sweeteners. For a number of reasons, these are worse for your health than ordinary sugar. So, if you drink diet soda regularly, you are at a higher risk of developing both cancer and diabetes.

- **Non-organic strawberries**

Some fruits and vegetables contain so many toxins from pesticides and fertilizers, that they are actually dangerous to eat. One of them is strawberries. Besides the pesticides, the soil on which non-organic strawberries are grown, is often treated with toxic gases. These were initially developed for chemical warfare but are now used in agriculture. In other words, if you can't afford organic strawberries, stay away from them.

CHAPTER 11

Approved Foods

We have seen how this diet can help us. Let's see what foods we can use to obtain the best results.

The nutritional plan of this diet is a very strict one. What is not on the list, you should avoid as much as possible!

- **Vegetables**

Vegetables are parts of plants consumed by humans as food. They are mostly low in fat and starches but high in minerals, vitamins, and dietary fiber. Any nutritionist will encourage you to consume at least five portions of vegetables a day.

Vegetables have an important effect on the acidic-alkaline balance.

The vegetables for the Dr. Sebi Diet are:

- **Asparagus**

Asparagus is an ancient plant, low in calories and sodium, but rich in vitamins, dietary fiber, folic acid, potassium, and chromium- a mineral that regulates the ability of insulin to transport glucose from the bloodstream to the cells.

Water makes up 93% of its composition; therefore, it's also used for diuretic properties.

It can be eaten raw- in salads, stir-fried, grilled, or in soups. In soups, it looses most of its nutrient properties.

This rule stands for any food that is boiled or over steamed. Raw foods, as Dr. Sebi says, are the best choice of nutrition. Other nutritionists apply the same rule to their diets.

- **Amaranth**

Amaranth can be used as a leaf vegetable or as grains. We will use both for our diet!

It is rich in carbohydrates, dietary fiber, minerals, and proteins. It is low in fat and does not contain gluten.

Stir-fried, steamed, or raw the best way to consume it. Grains can be eaten cooked or ground into flour for cookies, cereals, bread, crackers, and other baked products.

- **Avocado**

The avocado has American origins and is rich in vitamins, carotenoids, and fats. It is common in any vegetarian diet as a substitute for meat just because it has a high fat content.

Generally, avocado is served raw, but it is also used for juices and soups.

- **Bell peppers**

Bell peppers (red, green, white, purple, or yellow) are some of the sweetest vegetables.

They are native to Central America, Mexico, and northern South America but are now cultivated worldwide.

They are high in water (94%), vitamins, and carbohydrates and low in fat and proteins.

Served mostly raw, they make an exquisite and eye-catching dressing for green salads and sandwiches. Stir-fried, grilled, and steamed are also good ways to enjoy these tasty vegetables.

- **Cucumbers**

An ancient vegetable with mild melon flavor and slightly bitter taste.

Cucumbers are high in water (95%), vitamins, and kilocalories, but are low in essential nutrients.

We must eat it raw for this diet because pickled cucumbers contain acidic additives and sugar, which we must keep at bay.

- **Chickpeas aka Garbanzo beans**

Chickpeas are used in salads, soups, hummus (the main ingredient), and ground into flour.

They are an ancient plant, rich in proteins, dietary fiber, minerals, vitamins, and essential amino acids. They are 60% water and low in fat.

They are generally served rapidly boiled for 10 minutes and then simmered for a long time. It is used in salads, soups, ground into flour, and as an ingredient for veggie burgers, just like amaranth grains, both delicious and nourishing.

- **Chayote**

Chayote is an edible plant with American origins, rich in vitamins and amino acids.

It can be eaten raw, in salads and salsas, cooked just like the summer squash, or stir-fried.

Generally, we eat the fruit, but in some countries, shoots and leaves are also used for salads or stir-fries.

In the Dr. Sebi diet, it is used due to its diuretic and anti-inflammatory properties. The tea made of Chayote leaves is used to treat hypertension, dissolve kidney stones, and treat arteriosclerosis.

These are essential properties for detoxifying our bodies.

- Dandelion greens

Dandelion is native to North America, and Eurasia used as food and medicine.

It is high in vitamins and minerals. It contains 86% water, carbohydrates, moderate amounts of proteins, and very low fat.

The entire plant is edible, but we will use only the leaves. They have a bitter taste, but they make an exquisite ingredient for our green salads.

In the Mediterranean area is the most common ingredient of all diets, mainly for losing weight.

It is rich in calcium, so it's essential for the growth and strength of bones. Dandelion also helps the liver functioning, protect it from aging, and treat liver bleeding.

It has been used in traditional medicine in China, America, and Europe. Dandelion is good for liver disorders, urinary disorders, diabetes, anemia, jaundice, and some types of cancer.

The dandelion powder is used to increase urine production and as a laxative. It is the ultimate skin toner, blood tonic, and digestive tonic.

It contains alkaline chemicals that make it a great anti-inflammatory agent. Some people use it for loss of appetite, joint pain, bruises, upset stomach, and gallstones.

- Kale

Kale or leaf cabbage has Mediterranean and Asian origins and has been cultivated for food for centuries.

It is high in carbohydrates, vitamins, dietary minerals, carotenoids, and low in proteins and fat. It is composed of 84% water and can be eaten raw, stir-fried, or steamed.

Stir-frying or steaming because it reduces the levels of glycosylate compounds, which are potentially dangerous for our health. For now, research has not yet shown that it affects our health.

All we know so far is that kale is included in any diet, prescribed by nutritionists or not. Mediterranean diet, the Sirtfood diet, and even Dr. Sebi's diet.

Kale is a tasty ingredient to salads, veggie burgers, pasta, and smoothies.

- **Lettuce**

Lettuce is a leaf vegetable originally farmed by ancient Egyptians used for food and medicine.

Generally eaten raw, lettuce is a good source of vitamins, beta-carotene, folate, and iron.

It was used in medicine for typhoid, smallpox, rheumatism, nervousness, and coughs, but no scientific evidence has been found so far.

- **Mexican squash**

The Mexican squash is a vegetable used for food in soups, pickled, fried, grilled, in pasta, on pizzas, and even raw- in salads, sliced or shredded.

It has a low content in kilocalories but is high in folate, potassium, and vitamins.

- **Mushrooms (except for Shiitake)**

The mushroom is the fleshy fruiting body of a fungus. They are high in water (92%), carbohydrates, and vitamins but low in proteins and fat.

Edible mushrooms are used in cuisine all over the world for their delicious taste. Pay attention to toxic or hallucinogenic mushrooms!

They are used in traditional Chinese medicine, even if there is no evidence of benefits for health.

- **Onions**

Onions are vegetables with ancient Asian origins used as food and as medicine. They are used for healing oral sores, sleep disorders, ocular ailments, lumbago, and dysentery. It is one of the most worldwide known natural antibiotics.

They are about 89% water, rich in carbohydrates, and low in dietary fiber, proteins, and fat.

- **Okra**

Okra is an edible seed pod with Asian or South African origins, rich in carbohydrates, vitamins, dietary fiber, and low in proteins and fat.

For our diet, we may use both the leaves and the seeds. When the seed pods are cooked, it results in a slime, and that paste contains soluble fiber. To "deslime" it, you should use an acid, so it's best to eat it raw or included in salads since we want to maintain an alkaline state of our body.

Okra is high in water (90%), carbohydrates, vitamins, and folate and low in proteins and fat.

We can also consume its leaves and seeds.

- **Olives**

The olive is an ancient tree, and its fruits are the core ingredient of the Mediterranean cuisine.

In our diet we can use olives and olive oil, a must in any diet.

The olives are a significant source of calories, vitamins, and water (75%) but are low in proteins and carbohydrates.

- **Purslane**

Purslane, aka duckweed, is a vegetable with European and North African origins that can be eaten raw, stir-fried, cooked, or in soups and stews.

It is high in water (93%), carbohydrates, calcium, and magnesium, relatively high in vitamins, but low in fat and proteins.

- **Squash**

The squash has Central American origins, and only five species are grown for their edible fruits and seeds.

Raw squash is 94 % water. It is a rich source of nutrients, such as vitamins and dietary minerals. It is low in proteins and fat.

The seeds contain vitamins, saturated oils, and fatty acids.

It is a flavorful ingredient for desserts, puddings, biscuits, salads, soups, bread, and the famous pumpkin pie.

It's best to eat it raw, but stir-fried or gently steamed works too.

- **Sea vegetables aka seaweeds**

(Kelp/Dulse/Nori/Wakame)

Seaweeds are marine algae with the vital role of producing up to 90 % of Earth's oxygen. Only some species are edible.

They can be used for desserts, beverages, salad dressings, sauces, baked products. They are great dietetic foods.

In medicine, they are used because they keep at bay some DNA and RNA-enveloped viruses. The pills made from seaweed extract have the same effect of the gastric banding- they expand in the stomach to make it feel full.

- **Tomatoes (Cherry and Plum only)**

Tomatoes are some of the tastier vegetables on Earth, with South American origins. Even if they have the sweetest taste, tomatoes can be quite acid too, so Dr. Sebi suggested using only cherry and plum varieties for our diet. In this way, we won't be eating more acidic foods than we need.

They are a moderate source of vitamins but are low in carbohydrates, proteins, and fat. They are 95% water.

- **Tomatillo**

The tomatillo, aka the Mexican husk tomato, is similar to tomatoes. It has the same water content (95%); it is high in vitamins and low in proteins and fat.

They are eaten raw or cooked in lots of dishes, particularly salsa verde, but also soups, salads, stir-fries, and desserts. They can also be dried for an enhanced sweetness of the fruit. Raw, purple, or green tomatillo turns into a vary flavorful and eye-catching dressing for green salads.

- **Turnip greens**

Turnip is a vegetable with ancient Greek and Roman origins. We can eat the leaves and the roots.

The leaves and roots are 93% water, a rich source of vitamins, and low in carbohydrates, proteins, and fat.

They make an excellent garnish for green salads or any other dish if stir-fried or gently steamed.

- **Watercress**

Watercress is an aquatic plant, grown worldwide for its spicy leaves.

The leaves contain 95% water and significant amounts of vitamins, but they are low in dietary fiber, carbohydrates, proteins, and fat.

It's for the best to consume it raw or stir-fried, if boiled or steamed, it loses all its nutrient properties.

- **Wild arugula**

Arugula, aka rocket, is from the mustard family, with European and Asian origins. It grows wildly in temperate climate areas.

Arugula is 92% water, it is high in vitamins, carotenoids, polyphenols, and ascorbic acid, but low in proteins and fat.

It has a spicy, pungent flavor that makes it the best choice for green salads. Consume it only raw or stir-fried; if not, it will lose all its properties and distinguished taste.

It is a great ingredient for pizzas, pasta dishes, or soups.

In medicine, it is used for the treatment of gastroenteritis and the regulation of the intestinal transit.

- **Zucchini**

The zucchini is the Italian variety of squash, cultivated for the first time in the 19th century.

It is high in potassium, vitamins, and folate but low in proteins and fat.

It can be eaten raw (sliced or shredded), steamed, grilled, stir-fried, and cooked in several dishes. It's a tasty addition to green salads. It can also be pickled, but that is not good for our diet since pickles contain acid additives.

CHAPTER 12

Approved Fruits

Fruits are also a gift from Mother Nature. They are a significant source of food for humans. Except for their sweet taste (they are relatively high in sugar), they also contain fibers, water, and vitamins.

They are also a great stimulus for stomach secretions and appetite. Fruits are also helpful for the drainage of the liver and digestive tract, having a significant influence on the peristalsis to evacuate the intestinal content and prevent constipation.

The fruits for the Dr. Sebi Diet are:

- **Apples**

Apples are fruits with ancient Asian origins, now cultivated worldwide.

It is high in water (86%), a moderate source of dietary fiber, carbohydrates, and has a low content of micronutrients, fat, and proteins.

It is used for desserts, juices, or baked products.

- **Bananas**

Bananas are one of the sweetest fruits on Earth, with Austronesian origins, introduced to the Americas in the 16th century. The good news is that they are available year-round.

They are quite high in water (75%), potassium, vitamins, and carbohydrates, a moderate source of dietary fiber, and low in proteins and fat.

Generally, it is eaten raw but is also used for smoothies, desserts, or cooked, deep-fried, baked, steamed, or ground into flour.

- **Cherries**

Cherries have been consumed since prehistoric times in Europe, Asia, and North Africa. They were introduced in the Americas in the 15th century.

Sweet cherries are 82 % water, are a moderate source of carbohydrates, vitamins, and dietary fiber, and are low in proteins and fat. Sour cherries, instead contain more vitamins and beta-carotene.

They can also be used for beverages and desserts.

- **Cantaloupe**

Cantaloupe, aka sweet melon, has Asian origins, now spread worldwide.

It is 90% water, rich in vitamins, low in carbohydrates, proteins, and fat.

The fruit is eaten raw, in salads, or as dessert. The seeds are also edible. Dried and gently baked, they make an excellent snack.

- **Cactus fruit**

Cactus fruit, commonly called prickly pear, is spread throughout the Americas, in various species.

It has 88% water, a moderate source of carbohydrates, dietary minerals, and vitamins, low in proteins and fat.

It is used for salads, soups, desserts, beverages, candy, and drinks.

In medicine, it is used for open wounds as a coagulant and for the treatment of inflammation of the urinary and digestive tracts.

Research has shown that it aids in the prevention of diabetes, metabolic syndrome, obesity, cardiovascular disease, and some cancers.

So, there is a reason for Dr. Sebi's choice in using this fruit. It was also shown that consumption of cactus fruit leads to a reduced body circumference and BMI (body mass index).

- **Currants**

The currants are grown for their edible berries. Ribes and black currants are the best choices for our diet.

They have European and Asian origins, and are 82% water, a rich source of carbohydrates, iron, and vitamins, and are low in proteins and fat. Their seeds are rich in unsaturated fatty acids.

In medicine, they are used for the treatment of kidney diseases and for menstrual and menopausal problems.

- **Dates**

Dates have ancient Northern African origins, introduced into Mexico and California in 1765. Medjool dates are the best choice for any diet, including ours.

Dates can be eaten raw or cooked for various desserts and puddings. They can be stir-fried, dehydrated, ground into flour, or as juice.

They have a sugar content of 80 % and are a moderate source of proteins, fiber, potassium, manganese, selenium, and zinc.

Research on mice has shown that the aqueous extract of date seeds reduces DNA damage.

- **Figs**

Figs are native to Asia and the Mediterranean region.

The fruits contain monosaccharide sugars and mixed phytochemicals, such as flavonoids, rutin, and chlorogenic acid. Dried fruits contain higher levels of sugar and polyphenols.

- **Mango**

Mango is a juicy fruit, native to South Asia, now worldwide spread.

It is a rich source of vitamins, folate, and other nutrients. It contains carotenoids and polyphenols.

It can be eaten raw as a fruit, in juices, and ice cream, pickled, or cooked, in pies and sauces.

- **Oranges**

Oranges are native in Asia, introduced into the Americas in the 15th century, and can be eaten fresh, processed for juice, oils, and marmalade.

They are rich in vitamins, carotenoids, flavonoids, and various volatile organic compounds.

- **Papayas**

Papayas are originated in Central America and can be eaten raw only if peeled or cooked. The black seeds are also edible and have a spicy taste.

They contain 88% water, are a significant source of vitamins, folate, and carbohydrates but are low in proteins and fat.

It has been used in traditional medicine to treat malaria, relieve asthma, or as a purgative. All these uses make it a great choice for our diet, according to Dr. Sebi.

- **Plums**

Plums are fruits related to peaches and cherries. They have ancient European and Asian origins with a large variety of species.

They are 87% water, a moderate source of vitamins and carbohydrates but low in fat and proteins.

In medicine are used as a purgative, it works just fine for the regulation of the intestinal tract.

- **Pears**

Pears have been used since prehistoric times. Their origins are Chinese and are used raw, canned, in juices, or dried.

A pear is 84% water, it is a moderate source of carbohydrates, vitamins, and dietary fiber, but contains low levels of proteins and fat.

- **Peaches**

Peaches are also native to China, was introduced into the Americas in the 16th century, and is probably the juiciest fruit.

They are 89% water, a moderate source of carbohydrates and essential nutrients, but are low in calories, proteins, and fat.

They are rich in polyphenols, rutin, and chlorogenic acid.

- **Prunes**

Prunes are dried plums. They are 31% water, a rich source of carbohydrates, dietary minerals, and vitamins, but very low in proteins and fat.

- **Seeded grapes**

Grapes are delicious, juicy fruits with Eastern origins, cultivated for fruits or for making wine, jam juices, vinegar, and grape seed oil.

Grapes are 81% water, a moderate source of carbohydrates, vitamins, and calories, but low in fat and proteins.

The grape seeds contain healthy omega-3 fatty acids and twice the content of polyphenols of grape skins. They are packed with highly concentrated nutrients and vitamins. So, for our diet, we must use only seeded grapes.

They are useful for heart and brain health and are beneficial to the skin.

- **Seeded key limes**

Key limes are valued for their unique flavor. They are native to Southeast Asia, now worldwide spread.

Limes are 88% water, a rich source of vitamins, a moderate source of carbohydrates and polyphenol, but very low in fat and proteins.

Seeds are richer in vitamins and lower in acids.

We can eat them fresh as a fruit or juices, or dried as a flavor for exotic recipes, especially desserts.

- **Seeded melons**

Melons are juicy, sweet, and fleshy fruits, with Central American origins and with a large variety of species.

They are high in vitamins and short in proteins and fat. They have a high content in natural sugar.

- **Seeded raisins**

Raisins or dried grapes are the best of choices for tasty snacks.

They are useful for heart and brain health and are beneficial to the skin.

- **Soft jelly coconuts**

Soft jelly coconuts are fruits grown all throughout Jamaica; the edible part inside is usually called jelly.

It is a significant source of dietary fiber, but it is low in proteins, carbohydrates, and fat.

It can be used on its own and as an ingredient for salads, desserts, and drinks.

It is used for the regulation of the digestive systems and detoxifying internal organs

- **Sour soups (European or Asian markets)**

Sour soups are used in Eastern Europe and Asian cuisine for their sour taste.

They mainly contain natural ingredients with a slightly acidic flavor.

- **Tamarind**

Tamarind has African origins and produces pod-like fruits with sweet and tangy pulp.

It is a significant source of vitamins, sugar, calcium, and tartaric acid.

Some consider the fruit too sour but is used for many savory dishes.

In medicine, it is used for its laxative effects and as a poultice for patients with fever.

Research has shown that it has antioxidant properties, and that is helpful in liver diseases, for the coagulation system and antimicrobial response.

Grains

As I mentioned above, only whole grains are best, not refined ones. They are rich in carbohydrates, nutrients, and dietary fiber.

You are permitted to eat grains in the form of pasta, cereal, flour, or bread.

For the Dr. Sebi Diet, the approved grains are:

- **Amaranth**

Amaranth grains are a rich source of dietary minerals, a moderate source of proteins and carbohydrates, and very low in fat.

- **Fonio**

Fonio is a notable crop, mainly cultivated in West African countries, aka "hungry rice".

The grains are used for foods and beer.

They are highly nutritious, gluten-free, and rich in dietary fiber.

- **Kamut (Khorasan wheat)**

Kamut is the Oriental variety of wheat. It has Oriental origins and a rich, nutty flavor.

It is highly nutrient; it is a moderate source of proteins, dietary fiber, vitamins, and minerals but is low in fat.

The only bad news is that it contains gluten, so it's unsuitable for people with gluten-related disorders.

- **Quinoa**

Quinoa is part of the amaranth family with origins in South America.

It is high in carbohydrates, folate, and dietary minerals, a moderate source of proteins, vitamins, and low in fat.

Quinoa is gluten-free.

- **Rye**

Rye is a grass grown for its grains, with ancient Eastern origins, used for flour, bread, and alcoholic drinks.

It is rich in carbohydrates, dietary fiber, and vitamins but low in proteins and fat. It also has a low content of gluten, so it is unsuitable for people with gluten-related disorders.

In medicine, it is known for the regulation of blood sugar and the improvement of cholesterol levels.

- **Spelt**

The spelt is just another variety of wheat, an ancient crop throughout Europe, introduced into the States only in the 19th century. Now it has found a new market as a "health food".

It is a significant source of proteins, dietary fiber, vitamins, and carbohydrates.

Unfortunately, it also contains gluten, therefore a problem for those suffering from gluten-related disorders.

It is generally used as flour for baked products and is very easy to find in bakeries.

- **Teff**

Teff is another African grass, cultivated for its edible seeds.

It is a significant source of carbohydrates, proteins, dietary fiber, and manganese but low in fat.

It is gluten-free and can be used as flour for bread, other baked products, and alcoholic drinks in the Ethiopian culture.

- **Wild rice**

Wild rice is a semi-aquatic plant that was historically eaten in China and North America.

It is a moderate source of proteins, amino acids, and dietary fiber but is low in vitamins, iron, potassium, and fat. It contains no gluten.

The grains can be stewed or steamed.

Nuts and seeds

Nuts and seeds are energy-dense and nutrient-rich foods. For our diet, the approved nuts and seeds are:

- **Brazil nuts**

The Brazil nut is a South American tree, notable for its high content in selenium, which is responsible for the increase of HDL (good cholesterol).

It is also s a rich source of proteins, omega-6 fatty acids, dietary fiber, vitamins, and minerals.

- **Hemp seed**

Hemp is one of the first plants to be cultivated in Asia and Europe. It was introduced into the Americas in the 15th century.

Hemp seeds can be eaten raw, ground into dried powder, or as a liquid for beverages.

In the US, hemp seeds are used legally in food products, as of 2000.

They are high in calories, proteins, dietary fiber, vitamins, iron, zinc, and fat but low in carbohydrates.

When it comes to the protein level that hemp ensures us, it is considered a good substitute for meat, milk, eggs, and soy.

- **Raw sesame seeds**

Sesame is one of the oldest oilseed crops known, with Indian origins, notable for its rich and nutty flavor. It is one of the most used spices in cuisines all around the world.

Sesame seeds are high in carbohydrates, fat, vitamins, and dietary minerals. They are low in proteins.

In medicine, sesame consumption leads to small reductions in systolic and diastolic blood pressure, oxidative stress markers, and lipid peroxidation.

- **Raw sesame "Tahini" butter**

Tahini is a condiment made from toasted or raw sesame seeds. Raw Tahini is sold as an organic food product.

Mostly used in the Eastern, Mediterranean, and North African cuisine, it's a rich source of dietary minerals, calcium, and proteins.

It makes a useful addition in any vegetarian and vegan diets, and especially in ours, when eaten raw.

- **Walnuts**

The walnuts have been used in cuisine all over the world for centuries. Eaten raw or toasted, they make a popular addition to savory dishes, desserts, or for alcohol drinks in some countries.

They have a savory flavor, which makes them an interesting dressing for salads.

They are high in fat, carbohydrates, dietary minerals, and vitamins. They are a moderate source of proteins and dietary fiber.

Non conclusive research claimed that consumption of walnuts reduces the risk of coronary heart disease. The thing we know for sure is that walnuts are brain food and somewhat natural antibiotic.

In alternative medicine, walnuts are used to treat some heart diseases and even cancer, but there is no scientific evidence.

Dr. Sebi claimed it heals Candida because it kills all parasites.

Walnut hulls powder is used for healthy digestion and bowel regularity. It is also a powerful detoxifier, and it helps us balance the blood sugar levels.

Oils

Edible oils are rich in proteins and alkaloids. They are used for various purposes in food preparation and in cooking.

For our diet, the approved oils are:

- **Avocado oil**

Avocado oil is an edible oil used as an ingredient in all sorts of dishes or as cooking oil. It does not derive from seeds but from the fleshy pulp of the fruit.

It is high in vitamins, carotenoids, and unsaturated fats. It is naturally low acidic, which makes it a good choice for Dr. Sebi's diet. We can use it to stir fry, deep fry, grill, and sauteing our foods.

- ## Coconut oil (uncooked)

Coconut oil is an edible oil derived from the kernel or meat of mature coconuts.

It is high in fatty acids, that's why we are advised to limit somewhat the consumption. FDA and other health organizations draw attention to the increased risk of cardiovascular diseases and weight gain due to the high caloric properties of this oil.

In fact, clinical trials have shown that consumption of coconut oil leads to increased levels of LDL (bad cholesterol), so it should not be viewed as a healthy oil.

Only RBD (refined, bleached, and deodorized) coconut oil can be used as a cooking oil.

- ## Grapeseed oil

Grapeseed oil is made of pressed seeds. It may be used as cooking oil, salad dressing, a base for oil infusions of herbs and spices, and in baked products.

It is relatively high in polyphenols, fatty acids, and low in vitamins and saturated fats.

There is no scientific evidence of health benefits.

- ## Hemp seed oil

The hemp seed oil is obtained from pressed seeds. It is high in omega-3 and omega-6 fatty acids, and it is a moderate source of unsaturated and saturated fat.

It is not suitable for frying but can be used as a food oil or dietary supplement.

- ## Olive oil (uncooked)

Olive oil is obtained from pressed olives and is one of the essential ingredients of the Mediterranean cuisine.

It is used as cooking oil, but in our diet, we must only use it uncooked, so we make the most of its properties. It is the perfect addition to green salads and an additive for all sorts of dishes.

It is relatively high in fatty acids, very low in proteins and fiber, and is naturally low acidic.

There is no scientific evidence of its health benefits so far.

- **Sesame oil**

Sesame oil is an edible oil that can be used as cooking oil or as a flavor for all sorts of dishes, due to its nutty taste.

It is relatively high in fatty acids, vitamins, and calories.

In alternative medicine, is used for getting rid of fever. Studies have been made to attest to the effect on inflammation and atherosclerosis but with no conclusive results.

CHAPTER 13

Approved Herbs

Herbal teas

H erbs are used since ancient times as medicines and for a good reason. They work! They are plants with savory or aromatic properties that are used for flavoring foods or as teas- as a source of relaxation or for medical purposes.

Herbal teas contain caffeine- a stimulant of the CNS (central nervous system), tannins with an astringent effect, and mineral salts.

In addition to teas, you are free to drink as much water as possible. This promotes the elimination of harmful elements from the organism and increases your weight loss.

Liquids ensure the liver's activity and, most importantly, diuresis.

Remember to use pure water, as much as possible!

For the Dr. Sebi Diet, the approved herbal teas are:

- **Anise**

Anise is a spice with Eastern origins, grown mainly for its seeds.

It is high in proteins, also relatively high in fatty acids and dietary fiber.

Tea from whole or ground seeds, alone or combined with other herbs, is considered a regulator of digestion. It also has diuretic properties and can be used as a tranquilizer or to help people who suffer from insomnia.

- **Burdock**

Burdock is native to Europe and Asia, notable for its sweet yet pungent flavor, similar to an artichoke.

The whole plant can be eaten, but we will use tea from dried leaves.

It is high in dietary fiber, calcium, and amino acids, but is low in calories.

In traditional medicine is used as a diuretic and blood purifying agent. It also lowers the cholesterol level, and it stimulates the liver's functioning.

Burdock roots are used for acne, psoriasis, and carbuncles because it kills fungus and bacteria. It can also be used as a diuretic and detoxifier of the skin.

- **Chamomile**

Chamomile is an ancient plant that grows wildly in most countries.

Its flowers are high in polyphenols and essential oils.

In traditional medicine, it is used for the treatment of insomnia. Clinical studies have shown no evidence of its potential anti-anxiety properties so far.

Its anti-inflammatory properties are efficient in digestive system disorders, stomach ulcers, and colic.

Chamomile tea is a great antiseptic and has an anti-inflammatory effect. It is also used to calm the central nervous system, treat ADHD, fibromyalgia, hay fever, nervous asthma, and other sleep disorders.

- **Elderberry**

Elderberry is grown for its berries, leaves, and flowers.

It is high in water (80%), carbohydrates, vitamins but low in calories, proteins, and fat.

In medicine, elderberry tea is used as a dietary supplement for the treatment of colds, flu, and constipation. It's the number one enemy of mucus buildup.

It is also helpful in boosting the immune system; that's why Dr Sebi claimed it could cure AIDS. Back and leg pain, nerve pain, and chronic fatigue syndrome are just other disorders that elderberries can treat.

- **Fennel**

Fennel is an aromatic herb, worldwide grown for its edible leaves and fruits with a taste similar to anise.

It is high in dietary fiber, vitamins, and carbohydrates, but relatively low in proteins and fat. Its aroma derives from the high content of volatile oils and phytochemicals such as rosmarinic acid and luteolin.

It can be used as a vegetable, as a spice, and as aromatic tea (from dried leaves or seeds).

In traditional medicine has been used since ancient times as a diuretic.

- **Ginger**

Ginger is a fragrant spice with Asian origins, grown for its flavorful roots. It can be used as a medicine, as vegetable, juice, and alcoholic drinks.

Ginger is 79 % water, is a moderate source of carbohydrates, vitamins, and dietary minerals, but is low in proteins and fat.

Ginger herb tea is used for keeping at bay nausea that results from chemotherapy or pregnancy. It is also used for its anti-inflammatory properties and to relieve pain in osteoarthritis. So far, there is no clear evidence of those effects.

- **Red raspberry**

Red raspberry, aka European raspberry, is a sweet, edible fruit, also grown for its leaves.

The red raspberry is grown for its fruits, leaves, and roots.

It is a rich source of antioxidants, vitamins, potassium, iron, and magnesium, and the tea is used for killing stomach and colon cancer cells. Some research on mice have shown that red raspberry consumption prevented kidney stones formation. In medicine, it is also used as a skin-whitening agent.

Women use it for its beneficial effect on the reproductive system, to alleviate nausea, leg cramps, and to improve sleep during the pregnancy. It also has effects on the uterus and pelvic muscles, leading to shorter and easier labors.

- **Tilia**

Tilia, aka basswood, is an ancient tree famous for its flowers and blossoms, which are very popular in traditional medicine, both in Europe and North America.

It has a very flavorful taste due to the volatile oil that it contains. It is used for its antioxidant and astringent properties.

The tea from leaves and flowers is used for colds, flu, infections, fever, high blood pressure, and migraines. It is also used as a sedative, antispasmodic, and diuretic.

 The tea from wood pieces is used for the treatment of intestinal disorders, for the protection of the liver, and in gallbladder disorders, and infections like cellulitis or ulcers of the lower leg.

Spices

Spices are parts of a plant used for flavoring our foods. They are sometimes used in medicine. They are low in calories, fat, proteins, and carbohydrates but rich in micronutrients, minerals, and vitamins. They also have antioxidant properties.

The convenient aspect of using spices in a diet is that they are the main "excitors" of the digestive secretions.

For our diet, the spices we have to use are:

- **Achiote**

Achiote is a South American tree, used as a spice and a natural dye to color foods, soaps, cosmetics, and pharmaceutical products.

It is high in beta-carotene, essential oils, vitamins, and fatty acids.

In traditional medicine, it has been used for centuries for its therapeutic properties.

- **Basil**

Basil is a culinary herb, with African and Asian origins. It has a distinct sweet yet pungent smell and taste.

It is high in essential oils and probably the most common spice in the entire world, used for all sorts of dishes and some drinks.

Just like achiote, it has been used in traditional medicine.

- **Bay leaf**

Bay leaf is just another popular spice, with various species and different flavors used in the cuisine worldwide.

It is relatively high in essential oils and lauric acid.

- **Cloves**

Cloves are the flower buds of an Indonesian tree, used as a spice in the Mediterranean, Asian, African, and Eastern cuisine.

It is high in essential oils, tannins, and oleanolic acid. It also contains some bioactive chemicals, which makes it a perfect insect repellent.

In traditional medicine, the essential oil has been used as an analgesic or in aromatherapy.

But there is no scientific evidence that it works as an analgesic for any pain, except for alveolar osteitis. It also lacks conclusive results from studies on fever or blood sugar levels reduction. In fact, the FDA has not approved its use for medical purposes because it may cause side effects in patients with liver disease, immune system disorders, and food allergies.

- **Cayenne**

Cayenne peppers are used a spice or herbal supplement, in its fresh form or as a dried powder.

- **Dill**

Dill is probably one of the most popular spices in all countries. It has Eurasian origins, grown for its leaves and seeds.

It is relatively high in carbohydrates, vitamins, and dietary minerals, but low in fat and proteins.

In traditional medicine, it has been used for its antibacterial properties.

- **Habanero**

Habanero is just another variety of chili peppers, with South American origins.

It is relatively high in carbohydrates and vitamins, but low in fat and proteins.

It contains capsaicin, a chemical used as an analgesic in dermal patches.

- **Oregano**

Oregano has Eurasian and Mediterranean origins, used as a spice, for its flavorful aroma. It is a core ingredient of Italian cuisine.

It is high in essential oils, carvacrol, and thymol.

- **Onion powder**

Onions are vegetables with Asian origins, now grown all around the world.

They are high in carbohydrates, vitamin C, calcium, and potassium. Low in fat and proteins, but contain fluoride.

It is considered a natural antibiotic.

Onion powder is dehydrated ground onion, used as a spice for all sorts of dishes.

- **Sage**

Sage is an herb with Mediterranean origins, now worldwide grown for its culinary and medicinal use.

In medicine, it is used as a pain reliever and for positive effects on the human brain.

- **Savory**

Savory is an herb with Mediterranean origins, used in cuisine and medicine.

It contains carvacrol, an antibacterial biochemical.

It has antiseptic, carminative, and digestive properties. It is used as a cure for colic, gastroenteritis, nausea, bronchial congestion, sore throat, and arthritis.

- **Thyme**

Thyme is an ancient herb, with European origins, used in cuisine and medicine for centuries.

It is high in essential oils, especially thymol.

In traditional medicine, it has been used for its antiseptic properties.

- **Tarragon**

Tarragon is an herb with Eurasian origins, now worldwide grown for medicinal and culinary uses.

It is high in phenylpropanoids, essential oils, and capillin, an antibacterial biochemical with potential anti-tumoral properties.

CHAPTER 14

Key Dr. Sebi Herbs

I n addition to the herbal teas mentioned above, Dr. Sebi gave us a list of the most used herbs for natural healing.

- **Sarsaparilla root herb**

Sarsaparilla is a plant with Central American origins, used as a base for a soft drink and root beer.

It contains iron, saponins, and beta-sitosterol, which has anti-inflammatory and liver-protecting properties.

It was used in traditional medicine to treat syphilis. Besides, it has diuretic and antibacterial properties, and it's an ultimate blood purifier.

Dr. Sebi said that it would cure anemia, impotence in men, herpes, and other STDs.

- **Yellow dock root herb**

Yellow dock is a flowering plant, with Eurasian origins. It is high in vitamins, iron, potassium, and oxalic acid.

We can eat the leaves- if not too mature because they become bitter, the seeds, and the roots.

It has been used in traditional medicine to cure anemia. It is a blood purifier and detoxifier, especially for the liver, but also for the gallbladder.

It stimulates bile production, therefore a better digestion. It stimulates bowel movement to help us eliminate the waste in the intestinal tract faster, and increases the frequency of urination to help us eliminate all toxins.

- **Bladderwrack**

Bladderwrack is a seaweed, discovered in 1811, and used for its high content in iodine. It is also high in beta-carotene, zeaxanthin, volatile oils, potassium, paste, and other minerals.

It should be avoided before surgeries because it has anticoagulant properties.

In traditional medicine, it is used to stimulate of the thyroid gland and as a treatment for cellulite and obesity. It can also be used to alleviate rheumatism and rheumatoid arthritis.

Bladderwrack powder is full of minerals that help our skin eliminate toxins, so we get rid of wrinkles, excess water retention, and dryness. It also helps us regulate thyroid function and reduce inflammation in joints.

- **Kelp**

Kelp is a seaweed, mostly encountered in Europe, Greenland, and North American coasts.

It is high in phlorotannins and iodine, relatively high in vitamins and dietary minerals.

It is used to regulate the thyroid's function. Kelp tea helps us remove mucus from our bodies. That's why Dr. Sebi advises us to use his organic kelp flakes.

Organic kelp granules help us stimulate the thyroid gland and control metabolism. We can also use them to strengthen our circulatory system, reduce the risk of strokes and heart diseases, ensure healthy bones and teeth. It is also helpful due to its cancer-fighting benefits.

- **Irish moss tea**

Irish moss is a species of red algae that grows on the coast of Europe and North America.

It is high in vitamins, minerals, and iodine. But low in fat and proteins. It is the only natural source of thyroid hormones and helps us eliminate the excess mucus in our body.

In traditional medicine, it is used to cure sore throat and chest congestion.

- **Sting nettle leaf**

Nettle leaf is a flowering plant with European origins, which has been used in traditional medicines for centuries.

It is relatively high in proteins, carbohydrates, and low in fat. It also contains a-linolenic acid (a valuable omega-3 acid).

In medicine was used since ancient times as a diuretic laxative. Now the plant is used as astringent, tonic, anti-rheumatic, anti-allergenic, decongestant, stimulant, kidney cleanser, and anti-spasmodic.

Some of the illnesses cured now are diabetes and cancer.

The sting nettle root in powder is an excellent blood purifier, diuretic, astringent for UTI (urinary tract infections), and kidney stones. It is also used for allergies, osteoarthritis, internal bleeding, anemia, diabetes, asthma, and lung congestion.

It is a remarkable tonic, also used for its anti-aging and wound healing properties.

- **Milk thistle**

Milk thistle is a plant with Eurasian origins, now encountered throughout the world.

It is a significant silymarin, which makes it the perfect plant for the liver's health. It can treat cirrhosis, hepatitis, gallbladder disorders, and jaundice. There is scientific evidence for the improved liver function and a decreased number of deaths in people with liver diseases after consumption of milk thistle.

- **Cleavers**

Cleavers has Eurasian origins, used for its edible leaves and seeds, but considered harmful in some places.

It is high in iridoid glycosides, alkaloids, flavonoids, citric acid, and coumarins.

In medicine, it is used as a diuretic and lymphatic tonic, therefore a valuable blood purifier. As a diuretic it helps us clean urinary stones and treat urinary infections.

Cleavers have a cleansing action for the lymphatic system, which helps us treat conditions like arthritis and psoriasis.

- **Wormwood**

Wormwood is a perennial plant with Eurasian and African origins, with a bitter taste, used as an ingredient for absinthe and other alcoholic drinks.

It is high in absinthin, essential oils, and lactones.

In medicine, it is used as a bitter tonic to ensure a healthy appetite, for dyspepsia, and various infectious diseases.

As the name shows, it has been used for centuries to expel tapeworms, threadworms, or roundworms.

- **Wild cherry**

Wild cherry is a tree from the Prunus family, with American origins.

Its fruits contain cyanogenic glycosides.

In traditional medicine, it was used to treat coughs and colds, alleviate pain and stimulate the digestive system. It was also used as a cure for bronchitis, fever, gout, and diarrhea.

- **Red clover**

Red clover is an herb with Eurasian origins, now grown all over the world, with edible leaves and flowers.

It is high in coumestrol and isoflavone. It can be used for cancer prevention, high cholesterol, cough, asthma, indigestion, STDs, and bronchitis.

It is best to avoid it in patients with coagulation disorders. It is considered a blood cleanser.

Women use it to alleviate symptoms of menopause, breast pain, and PMS (premenstrual syndrome).

Skin appliance is used for skin sores, burns, psoriasis, and some skin cancers.

- **Blue vervain**

Blue vervain is a herb, which naturally grows across North America.

It was used in traditional medicine for centuries, to stimulate the liver and other organs, and calm the central nervous system.

It is a tonic that can also be used to relieve respiratory congestion, ease coughs, lower fever, calm the nerves, and cleanse toxins.

- **Shepherd's purse**

It is a flowering plant from the mustard family, with Eurasian origins, used for food and medicine.

The shepherd's purse has antioxidant, anti-inflammatory, and anti-mucous properties. It is used as astringent in the infections of the urinary tract and also to reduce inflammation, protect us from ulcers, to stimulate circulation, and increase the flow of urine. We can use it to treat various diseases, such as bleeding disorders, diarrhea, bladder infections, low blood pressure, headaches, and kidney disease.

In the case of wounds and burns, it may be applied directly to the skin to soothe pain and promote healing.

There is little scientific evidence of its effect on slowing the growth of tumors.

- **Yarrow herb**

Yarrow herb is a flowering plant that grows in temperate regions with a long history of traditional medicine use.

It is high in essential oils, flavonoids, isovaleric acid, and salicylic acid.

It has been used for centuries in wounds repair in European and Asian traditional medicine. Native Americans used it for toothaches, to reduce fever, cure stomach ailments, and treat wounds and burns.

It is the ultimate herb for organ repair, and it can also be used in chronic diseases of the urinary tract, and as a tonic for the venous system and mucous membranes. It is efficient in sore throat, bleeding, incontinence of urine, and diabetes.

- **Chickweed**

Chickweed is a flowering plant with Eurasian origins, used for centuries as a herbal remedy.

It can also be used as a leaf vegetable, in salads or other dishes.

In traditional medicine, it has been used to treat itches, pulmonary diseases, rheumatic pains, and arthritis.

Now it is used as a diuretic and as demulcent since it alleviates the pain and inflammation of the mucous membrane by forming a soothing film over it.

Dietitians and herbalists use it because it suppresses appetite.

- **Valerian root**

Valerian is a flowering plant with European origins used in medicine since ancient times.

It is high in alkaloids, isovaleric acid, iridoids, and flavanones.

It is an effective sedative used to treat insomnia and other sleep disorders. It is also used for anxiety-related disorders, such as nervous asthma, fear of illness, and hysteria, but no study has shown conclusive results.

Some people use it to treat depression, mild tremors, ADHD (attention deficit-hyperactivity disorder), and CFS (chronic fatigue syndrome). Women also use valerian to soothe menstrual cramps, and to alleviate hot flashes and anxiety, both symptoms associated with menopause.

- **Damiana leaves**

Damiana is a Central American shrub with aromatic flowers and leaves with spicy smell and taste.

It is high in damianin, beta-carotene, flavonoids, glycosides, and relatively high in fatty acids and caffeine.

It is used in traditional medicine for increased energy, mild depression, menstrual pain, impotence, and sexual stimulation.

- **Chaparral**

Chaparral is a medicinal herb that grows across the Americas.

In traditional medicine, it has been used to treat STDs, tuberculosis, dysmenorrhea, chickenpox, and snake bites.

Now it is used to alleviate rheumatic and stomach pains, to treat bronchitis, arthritis, bowel cramps, colds, and chronic skin disorders.

It has also been used for stomach problems, gall bladder and urinary tract infections, kidney stones, and diarrhea.

Skin application is used for rheumatism, arthritis, minor wounds, back pain, and skin infections.

CHAPTER 15

Foods to Avoid

I n Dr. Sebi's Diet, some foods are not allowed, mainly processed foods, animal-based, or made with leavening agents. Some seedless fruits are also banned.

Because we have to deal with a diet, we must pay attention to certain supplements we will need. They range from vitamins and minerals to other nutrients, such as iron, calcium, and omega-3 fatty acids.

However, if you vary your meals often, you will get the most nutrients from the plant-based sources.

- **Sugar**

Instead of sugar, you should use sweeteners such as pure agave syrup (from cactus) or date sugar (from dried dates).

- **Salt**

Instead of refined salt, you may use the powdered, granulated seaweed or pure sea salt.

No GMO foods!

It is imperative to avoid pesticides and other chemicals added to processed foods or genetically modified ones. If it's not natural, it will harm us in the long-term.

The main foods to avoid are:

- **Meat of any kind**

Meat is a rich source of water (755), proteins, and vitamins, but is low in fat, carbohydrates, and dietary minerals. Even if the level of fat is low, depending on race, sex, age, and other factors, the negative aspect is that any meat contains cholesterol, which harms our overall health.

Nutritionists advise us to keep as far as possible from meat, especially the red one, because, for its consumers, there is a higher risk of cancer, heart diseases, and obesity.

Products made with processed meat is even worse, Dr. Sebi said. In addition to the high level of animal-based proteins, processed meat also contains food additives that will only increase the acidic state of our body.

- **Fish and seafood**

Fish and seafood are famous for the high content of omega-3 fatty acids, which are suitable for our brain, heart, and digestive system. Fish and seafood especially is a core ingredient of the Mediterranean diet. Still, we must keep in mind that it is also a relatively high source of damaging elements, such as marine toxins, microbes, pollutants, and other poisons, natural or human-made.

- **Dairy products**

Dairy products are used worldwide, in various forms and are harmful to people with lactose intolerance.

They contain cholesterol, calcium, and saturated fats that can lead to increased risk of heart disease, coronary artery calcification, and other problems.

Despite some wrong belief, milk and other dairy products do not cause mucus production, therefore don't make asthma symptoms worse.

They are avoided by vegans, only for an ethical reason regarding how the animals are handled and how dairy products are produced.

- **Eggs**

Eggs are just another rich source of animal-based proteins. They are also high in fat, calcium, vitamins, water (75%), and cholesterol.

According to Dr. Sebi and most nutritionists, eggs should be avoided as much as possible. In almost any diet, egg consumption is reduced to a maximum of two eggs a week, but Dr. Sebi advises us to set them aside.

There is a higher risk of developing heart diseases, such as strokes, cardiovascular disease, coronary artery disease, myocardial infarction, and type 2 diabetes.

- **Wheat**

Wheat is a crop with Eastern origins, now worldwide cultivated for its seeds.

It is high in carbohydrates, folate, dietary minerals, and relatively high in proteins and selenium, but low in fat. It is used as the main ingredient for bread, crackers, pasta, breakfast cereals, cookies, and some alcoholic drinks.

Most nutritionists claim that a diet rich in grains, vegetables, and fruits is bound to help us maintain a healthy weight, decrease the risk of heart diseases and some types of cancer.

The main problem with wheat is that it contains high gluten levels, a severe problem for those who suffer from gluten-related diseases, not only bloating, but sometimes, even neurological disorders, fibromyalgia, inflammation, and psychological disturbances.

- **Corn**

Corn is a cereal grain with American origins, worldwide famous for its sweet taste, but most of all, for popcorn.

It is high in water (76%), carbohydrates, a moderate source of dietary fiber, minerals, but low in fat and proteins.

Dr. Sebi advises us to keep it at bay because it contains lipid transfer protein. This protein that causes allergic reactions, such as vomiting, diarrhea, swelling of mucous membranes, and sometimes asthma.

- **Garlic**

Garlic is a close relative of the onion, with Asian origins, with a long history of consumption as food and medicine. It is considered a natural antibiotic. It has been used in traditional medicine to treat arthritis, chronic cough, insect and snake bites, and antiseptic to prevent gangrene.

It contains polysulfides, saponins, and flavonoids. It is low in carbohydrates, vitamins, dietary fiber, proteins, and fat.

It is banned from our diet because its consumption may lead to gastrointestinal discomfort, dizziness, allergic reactions, sweating, and bleeding. It also contains selenium, an essential trace element, which is toxic if taken in excess.

- **Sugar**

Sugar is high in carbohydrates and low in fat, proteins, and dietary fiber.

Sugar is a refined food, commonly used as an additive to processed foods. It is also very damaging to health. Most nutritionists claim that its excessive use is most likely to create addiction.

We know that it is related to an increased risk of type 2 diabetes, tooth decay, obesity, metabolic syndrome, cardiovascular disease, and even dementia.

As I already mentioned, it's for the best to use only the natural sugar from fruits, vegetables, or agave syrup and date sugar.

- **Fast foods**

Fast foods are the most pleasant and easy to make foods, and let's admit, the ultimate eye-catching and mouth-watering kind of food. Especially in our modern, hectic times!

We are always in a hurry, always on the run through jobs, family, and other daily concerns. Most of us don't even have the time to enjoy at least three meals a day. You're lucky if you get to have dinner quietly, with your family or friends!

The solution? Fast food, of course. Junk food and nothing else, but what can we do to change that? It is hard to start improving your eating habits, especially when you have to, just like in our case: a diet!

I have to mention the right mindset and strong will again. Not just with a twist of your nose or a snap of your fingers. With lots and lots of patience, and the gradual introduction of healthy ingredients to your diet!

Unfortunately, fast foods are always linked to obesity, high cholesterol levels, and even depression. For good reasons!

- **Processed foods**

Processed foods are even worse. All sorts of additives are included to make them taste better, to be appealing to customers, easy to eat on the go, and for longer shelf life.

Another negative aspect is that they contain little or no whole food; they are only fortified with micronutrients.

In the long run, all these additives, sweeteners, processing acids, flavors, and preservatives will make it harder for our body to keep up with harmful elements.

The increased consumption of processed foods leads to a higher risk of developing chronic diseases, such as obesity, diabetes, heart disease, hypertension, and some cancers.

- **Seedless fruits**

Seedless fruits are all fruits that contain no mature seeds. They are commercially valuable because their consumption is easier.

This category includes watermelons, grapes, tomatoes, and citrus fruits.

- **Soy products**

Soy is a bean with Asian origins, with several uses. Soy products are divided into three categories: unfermented (soy milk), fermented (soy sauce, bean paste, and tempeh), and defatted soybean meal (soy flour from the material remaining after extraction of oil).

They are high in dietary minerals, vitamins, and phytic acid. They also contain high levels of proteins, carbohydrates, and fat.

There is no conclusive evidence of its effect on health or cancer risk. But the relatively high content of isoflavones in soy may be useful in the treatment of cardiovascular diseases.

Another negative aspect is that soy commonly causes allergy.

- **Poultry**

Poultry is a domesticated bird. We eat their eggs and meat.

The white meat is high in proteins and low in fat. I already explained why Dr. Sebi advises us not to eat no meat or eggs.

Any food with added vitamins and minerals

If the food is not naturally high in minerals and vitamins, it's not suitable to eat. Adding nutrients will not ensure any health benefit. Instead, it may lead to harmful effects due to overdosing of some vitamins and minerals.

All foods leavened with baking powder or with yeast

Baking powder and yeast are used all over the world to make dough for baked products.

The negative aspect is that they are highly acidic. So, it's best to avoid these foods.

- **Alcohol**

Alcohol is banned in all diets, except for the Sirtfood one. In that case, we can drink some red wine for its high resveratrol content.

Alcohol is high in sugars, and its consumption leads to liver diseases.

- **Canned fruits or vegetables**

Canned fruits and vegetables are processed foods. Due to preservatives and sugars added, they are no longer natural and have a lower content of vitamins and proteins.

CHAPTER 16

Alkaline Plant-Based Diet

The Health Benefits of Alkaline Plant-Based Diet

If you are a vegetarian, vegan, or aiming to move in this direction, the alkaline diet is ideal. While all dietary plans can be built on a strong foundation of vegetables and fruits, a plant-based diet is one of the best options for adhering to this way of eating. Not all vegan or plant-based diets are alkaline; a lot of foods that are free of animal products can be processed and contain acidic ingredients, though once digested, many "acidic" fruits and vegetables become alkaline. One of the most beneficial, nutrient-rich foods for an alkaline diet is soy. Soybeans (edamame beans) are a great snack on their own, as is tofu, tempeh, miso, and other soy-based foods. When choosing soy products, look for organic, natural options, and avoid preservatives as much as possible.

Why Choose a Plant-Based Diet?

There are many reasons for moving to a plant-based diet, from reducing meat in your diet overall, to implementing one or two "meat-free days" each week. If your current diet is very meat-heavy, this will take some major adjustment, so it is best to not make the switch from red meats to full veganism overnight. Veganism or vegetarianism works best when whole, natural foods are chosen instead of packaged or processed options. A lot of marketing is involved in promoting meat-free packaged snacks and condiments, though many of these may contain sugars, high amounts of sodium, artificial color, additives, and other ingredients that are unhealthy.

There is a lot of research to support a plant-based diet, and the high amount of alkaline in many fruits and vegetables means a good fit with the alkaline-based diet:

- The emphasis is on the whole, natural foods, which simplifies the process of shopping and selecting foods for your diet. This also makes meal preparation and planning much easier, as your focus will be on vegetarian-based eating, without meat as an option, and little or no dairy.

- A plant-based diet can help with weight loss, as vegetables and fruits are digested and used much more quickly than meat and dairy products. There are also fewer calories contained in vegetarian meals, even where the actual portion size is the same or similar to a meal, including meat.

- Meeting your goal weight is a great achievement, and maintaining weight is another task. This can be done much more effectively with plant-based eating, as there are not only restrictions on meat and dairy consumption, but on processed foods, which sometimes contain meat by-products (gelatin) and a high amount of preservatives and artificial flavors.

- Soy is a major staple of a plant-based diet. The amount of calcium, protein, iron, and nutrients in soy products is comparable to meat, and with a fraction of the calories and fat. Soy is also relatively inexpensive and easy to find in most grocery stores. Tofu, tempeh, and edamame beans are popular ways to enjoy soy in almost any type of meal.

- Enjoying a plant-based diet can reduce or eliminate food sensitivities to dairy and meat products, as these are no longer a part of the diet. Other food allergies or sensitivities may be less of a factor, once a more pH balance is established in your body, as digestion becomes easier and health improves overall.

- The health benefits of a plant-based diet, especially vegan, where all meat by-products and dairy foods are eliminated entirely are numerous. From improving heart health and cardiovascular function to preventing cancer, type 2 diabetes, and many other conditions. Prevention is a big factor in why choosing a plant-based diet, as many conditions and diseases can be avoided in the first place.

The Benefit of Soy in an Alkaline Diet

When it comes to soy, there are a lot of studies and findings that result in positive outcomes and benefits of eating soy on the dangers of increasing estrogen and the impact of this on your health. Overall, soy is a healthy option for any diet, especially for plant-based vegan diets that avoid all meat products. For people with allergies to soy and soy-based products, some alternatives can be used to adhere to a vegan meal plan successfully. For most people, soy is a good option with the following advantages:

1. High in protein. Soy can provide just as much, if not more, protein in your diet than meat. In combination with a balanced diet that includes fresh vegetables and fruits, your body will receive more than the required daily protein.

2. Low in cholesterol: Plant-based foods are low in cholesterol, saturated, and trans fats, which makes them a good choice for good cardiovascular function and a way to prevent heart disease.

3. High in fiber. Soy, like all vegetables and fruits, is very high in fiber. Not only will you meet your daily protein, calcium, and iron requirements by switching to soy from meat, you'll also receive a good dose of fiber with each serving, which increases metabolism and keeps weight at a healthy, manageable level.

4. Vitamin B12 and other nutrients considered only available in meat and meat-related products are also found in some soy products. Fermented soy, such as miso and tempeh, contain a sufficient amount of B12 to meet dietary requirements.

5. Vitamin D is often an ingredient in dairy milk, due to being fortified, though this can also be found in various soy products as well. While only a small amount of this vitamin is required, it's important that it's a part of your diet.

6. Soy products come in many forms, textures, and flavors. Soft tofu varieties, for example, can be used to create puddings, cakes, and smoothies. Firm tofu and tempeh can be marinated and fried, baked, or sautéed with any combination of vegetables and ingredients. Soymilk is a great alternative to dairy and can be used with cereals, in smoothies, milkshakes, and as a refreshing beverage.

7. Easy to digest. While some people have reported bloating and mild issues with digesting soy, in general, it's easy food for the body to digest and break down for nutrients.

Alternatives to Soy for a Plant-Based Diet

If soy-based foods are not an option for your plant-based diet, there are many alternatives to choose from. These foods contain high amounts of protein, calcium, and iron, which are found in meats and dairy products:

Coconut-cultured yogurt:

Similar to dairy yogurt, vegan, coconut-based yogurt is made by cultivating bacterial culture from coconut to make a product with the same texture, nutrients, and a similar flavor to dairy yogurt.

Vegan cheese:

Most varieties of vegan cheese are soy-based, though a growing number of plant-based cheeses are made from vegetables and vegetable oils. The benefits of vegan cheese include a similar taste and texture to regular, dairy cheese. Vegetable-based cheese, as opposed to soy-based products, tends to melt easier, which makes this variety a preferred option for vegan grilled cheese and Mac-and-cheese dishes.

Almond, cashew, and coconut milk:

There are many non-dairy milk alternatives available at nearly every grocery store and local restaurant. Almond milk is becoming nearly as popular as soymilk, as well as other nut-based kinds of milk, including cashew milk. Some varieties include a combination of almond and coconut milk, or cashew and almond, for a pleasant, nut-like taste that works well in recipes, smoothies, and with cereal. More people are ditching dairy milk and cream for non-dairy options for their coffee and tea as well. Other alternatives include hemp and rice milk.

Nut Butters:

Peanut, almond, and other nut kinds of butter are an excellent source of protein and energy. Just one or two spoons of these butters will provide a good boost of nutrients before a workout or an active day.

Other Soy Alternatives:

Nuts and seeds can be added to stir fry dishes and salads, instead of tofu and other soy foods to boost the protein and calcium content. Olive oil or coconut oil is both good alternatives for baking and cooking vegetarian dishes. Both oils have a neutral flavor that works well with any combination of ingredients.

Alkaline Fruits

Fruits are an excellent source of vitamins, fiber, and energy, with natural sugars that can easily replace the need for sweet snacks and processed foods. When we shop for fruits, we tend to choose from a small circle or group of fruits that we are familiar and comfortable with. The variety or limitations on what fruit we buy can depend on what's in season, how much of a budget we have to work with, and our cravings. Bananas, apples, oranges, and berries tend to be most popular, and for a good reason: they are delicious and easy to eat. Apples are best during autumn when they are in peak season and are available in many varieties that vary in texture, taste, and appearance. During summer months, it's the perfect time to enjoy fresh fruits, such as berries, bananas, and melons.

If you buy local, fresh fruits become less available during winter or colder seasons. Frozen fruits are another option to consider. They are just as healthy and more convenient, as they last longer and can be used at any time. Canned foods, even vegetables or fruits should be avoided, as they contain extra sodium and sugar, along with other additives.

Which Fruits are high in Alkaline?

All fruits have a significant amount of alkaline, which makes them all good choices for an alkaline diet. The amounts vary depending on which fruit, where alkaline is either low, moderate, or high. Some fruits that contain acidic properties will convert to alkaline once digested, like tomatoes and citrus fruits, while others contain a high amount of alkaline before consumption:

1. Blackberries, strawberries, and raspberries. Berries are a great choice in an alkaline diet, due to their high amount of vitamin C and antioxidants.

2. Nectarines, like peaches, are high in alkaline and make a great snack on their own, or in a fruit salad.

3. Watermelons are not only high in alkaline but also contain a good amount of potassium and fiber. They are an excellent choice for a snack and especially refreshing during the summer season when they are more readily available.

4. Apples have more of an amount of alkaline that's more moderate to high, though they contribute a lot of nutrients that make them a preferred snack any time of the year. They can be enjoyed raw, stewed, or baked for a variety of dishes. Apples are also naturally sweet, which makes them ideal for desserts.

5. Bananas are high in potassium, fiber, and pack a lot of energy into just one serving. In fact, one banana can provide up to 90 minutes of energy; an easy and quick snack before a workout, hike, or going cycling.

6. Cherries, similar to berries, are high in alkaline and fiber. They also promote regularity and a healthy metabolism.

Are there any fruits to avoid? With an alkaline diet, virtually all fruits are good options, which make the diet an easy process to follow.

CONCLUSION OF "THE DR. SEBI

APPROVED HERBS HANDBOOK"

The diet approved by Dr. Sebi also known as Alfredo Bowman has permitted certain food items that are 100% vegan and are not processed or modified. Dr. Sebi is not a professional or does not hold any degree but he claims himself to be a self-taught herbalist. However, following this diet can help prevent the diseases such as heart diseases, diabetes, kidney disorder or liver diseases. This diet can also be used to reduce weight and reverse or prevent the already mentioned health problems.

Detoxification and cleansing has several health benefits even if it has few disadvantages. Few of the advantages of this are, it keeps you healthy and physically fit, boosts immunity, improve the focus of the person. Other than that there are also natural methods of detoxification such as dry brushing, cupping, souping, exercising etc. By adapting this diet, one can have several health benefits that are shinier hair, healthy and clear skin, improved immunity and overall optimal health. Herbs and Food Recipe provides the individual with variety and versatility who is looking forward to follow the diet approved by Dr. Sebi. There are lot of combinations for the approved items that can be achieved and enjoyed.

INTRODUCTION OF "THE DR. SEBI

TREATMENTS AND CURES"

D r. Sebi's cure and treatment is based the human's body ability to self-heal. Biologists have already proven beyond a reasonable doubt that the human body has a tremendous capability to fight every kind of disease. Asides the damaging effect of environmental pollution, the drugs that we take for symptomatic relief and the junk food that we consume in large quantities contribute to the development of several chronic diseases, which are quickly becoming the leading cause of death in the Western world. Bad eating habits and reliance on drugs weaken the body's defenses and disease-fighting ability.

Dr. Sebi's cure is rooted in herbs and barks: the only way to enhance the body's immunity healthily and naturally. You should consider adhering to his principles and diet not only because of the health benefits, but for the general wellbeing it fosters. But first, let's examine what Dr. Sebi's cure and treatment is all about and then we can move on to how his herbal cure for diseases works.

This diet is entirely based on the principle of African biomineral balance and was developed using the research of the self-taught herbalist Alfredo Darrington Bowman, better known as Dr. Sebi.

He designed his diet for everyone who wants to cure or prevent chronic diseases and improve their general fitness, without relying on conventional western medicines.

According to Dr. Sebi, disease is the result of the formation of mucus in a particular place in the body. For example, a buildup of mucus in the lungs is pneumonia, while the extra mucus within the pancreas is diabetes.

He states that diseases cannot exist in an alkaline environment and start to appear as soon as your body becomes too acidic. Therefore, by strictly following his weight loss plan and using his exclusive dietary supplements and herbs, you are guaranteed to restore your body's natural alkaline environment and detoxify your disease-riddled body.

The weight loss program includes a specific list of daily vegetables, climaxes, grains, nuts, seeds, oils, and herbs. Since animal products are not approved, Dr. Sebi's Healthy Eating Plan is considered a vegan diet. Sebi said that in order for your body to heal on its own, you must constantly observe the diet, for the rest of your life.

Dr. Sebi, a herbal practitioner has used his alkaline herbs and diets to cure herpes and chronic diseases for many years and the testimonials of his patients, including some very high profile ones, can attest to that.

This book will provide you with the complete breakdown of the herbs that have been used by Dr. Sebi to cure various diseases, viruses and easy, step-by-step guides about the preparation and doses of the herbs.
It also includes the detoxification of the complete body organs, tissues, and cells, the herbs provided for detoxification, and how to start a holistic work on the body.

CHAPTER 17

Who is Dr. Sebi and His Philosophy

The man behind the Dr. Sebi Diet is Alfredo Bowman. He is a Honduran self-proclaimed herbalist and healer who uses food to improve health. Although he is already deceased, he has a number of followers in the 21st century. Because of his holistic approach, he has claimed to cure many kinds of diseases using herbs and a strict vegan diet. He has set up a treatment center in his home country before moving to New York City, where he has continued his practice and extended his clienteles from Michael Jackson, John Travolta, Eddie Murphy, and Steven Seagal, to name a few.

Although he calls himself Dr. Sebi, he does not hold any medical nor Ph.D. degree. Moreover, the diet has claimed to cure different conditions such as sickle-cell anemia, lupus, leukemia, and HIV-AIDS. This leds to a lot of issues,particularly that he was practicing medicine without a license and his exorbitant claims. While he was charged for practicing without a license, he was acquitted in the early 1990s due to a lack of evidence. However, he was instructed to stop making claims that his diet can treat HIV-AIDS. While there are controversies that surround his name, there are so many benefits of his alkaline vegan diet that it is still popular even to this date.

The Dr.Sebi Alkaline Eating Diet

Dr. Sebi believed that acidity and mucus could cause different types of diseases. For instance, the build-up of mucus in the lungs can lead to pneumonia. He noted that eating certain types of food and avoiding others like the plague can help detoxify the body. It can also bring the body to an alkaline state that can reduce the risk of developing many types of diseases.

By turning the blood alkaline, the cells can be rejuvenated and can easily eliminate toxins out. Moreover, he argues that diseases cannot exist in an environment that is alkaline. His principle of making the body more alkaline is what other plant-based diets are banking on.

This particular diet relies on eating a list of approved foods as well as the intake of certain types of supplements. For the body to heal itself, Dr. Sebi noted that this diet should be followed consistently for the rest of your life.

The Dr. Sebi Diet is plant-based, but unlike other plant-based diets, there are some differences in this diet to the plant-based diet in general. Here is a compiled list of what differentiates the Dr. Sebi Diet from a plant-based diet.

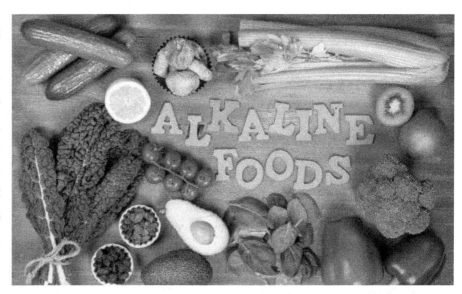

No processed foods: Tofu, veggie burgers, textured vegetable protein, canned fruits, canned vegetables, oil, soy sauce, and other condiments are considered processed. The Dr. Sebi Diet encourages dieters to consume food that is unadulterated. Some plant-based diets still allow the consumption of processed foods as long as they are made from plant-based ingredients.

No wheat products allowed: Under this diet regimen, you are not allowed to consume wheat and wheat products such as bread, biscuits, and others as they are not naturally growing grains. Naturally growing grains include amaranth seeds, wild rice, and triticale, to name a few.

The need to adhere to the food list: In general, plant-based diets are not so restrictive when it comes to the food that dieters are allowed to eat (unless you are specifically following a strict plant-based regimen such as the plant-based keto diet). However, the Dr. Sebi Diet requires dieters to only eat foods that are listed in the nutritional guide.

Drink one gallon of water daily: Water is the most hydrating liquid on the planet. The Dr. Sebi Diet requires dieters to consume 1 gallon of water daily or more. Moreover, tea and coffee should be avoided as these drinks are highly acidic.

Taking in Dr. Sebi's supplements: If you are taking any medications for a particular health condition, this particular diet regimen will require you to consume proprietary supplements an hour before taking your medication.

CHAPTER 18

Dr. Sebi Teachings and Methods

D r. Sebi proposed that the body is at the state of becoming susceptible to contracting diseases when the level of toxins and mucus accumulation increased.

He argued that people that are suffering from different diseases and those that are interested in preventing diseases should always eat an alkaline diet, bearing in mind that when the body removes the increased amount of acidic substances and mucus, it becomes free from infections.

He also suggested that cleansing and detoxification of the body is an essential and significant tool necessary in dealing with any form of the disease in the body.

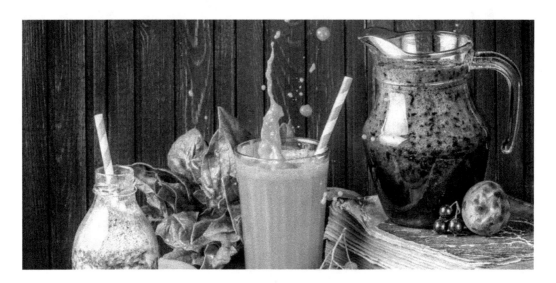

Detoxification of the body assists in the elimination of mucus accumulated in the liver, lungs, and many other body organs and also helps in the removal of excess acidic substances, thereby making the body free from disease-causing diseases.

Dr. Sebi also made use of herbs that are important in re-energizing and revitalizing the body. The organs of the body function properly when there is an improvement in your health, and this indicates that your body is void of diseases.

Dr. Sebi Classification of Food

Dr. Sebi classified food into six categories.
These categories are:

- Drugs.
- Genetically modified foods.
- Hybrid foods.
- Dead foods.
- Living foods.
- Raw foods.

He concluded that the first four categories of food in this list are no go area as they cause more damage in the body than good. These foods can cause a build-up of acids and mucus in the body. However, the last two categories of foods are the best types of food he classified as healthy because the nutritional contents in them are not lost in any way. For instance, foods that are thoroughly cooked, hybridized, and modified have lost the required amount of nutrients present in them. Hence, instead of providing benefits for the body, the reverse is the case. However, raw foods, especially vegetables, fruits, and herbs, are excellent for building good health.

Information about Dr. Sebi's Diet

Dr. Sebi's diets are diets that are plant-based and electric in nature. Dr. Sebi's diets are African bio-mineral diets which help dieters to fight diseases. The diet also serves as the prevention of various diseases (prophylaxis) and helps in boosting the immune system. When the body is immuno-compromised, it is said to accommodate any infection that sneaks in.

Dr. Sebi's diet is also beneficial for people who cherish to live a healthy life by remaining clean and lean. His diet was not created from heaven; they are common foods we ignore because of the love of modified, processed, refined, and hybridized foods.

Dr. Sebi's diet contains vegetables, fruits, grains, nuts, herbal teas, plant-based sweeteners, and seeds. Those who cherish animal products will not benefit from this diet as it does not encourage foods that are made from animals.

According to Dr. Sebi, all infections grow well in the environment that makes them comfortable such as acidic, mucus overload, and toxic environs.

When the body is in a limy condition, infections will find it so difficult to thrive, and when it is in an acidic state, the reverse is the case. Hence, the acidic component in the body helps diseases to multiply and thrive.

Likewise, he also declared that the build-up of excess mucus in the body increases the susceptibility of having an infection as the mucus block up the blood vessel and hinders the flow of blood easily.

He stated that the excess mucus must be removed for you to enjoy your health. When the mucus is removed either by detoxification or cleansing, the diseases are automatically removed.

The diets of Dr. Sebi have been proven effective by those who truly love them. The diets re-energize and revitalize the body by bringing it back to its normal state.

The healing of many sufferers who suffers from hair loss and many other prevalent diseases didn't occur because of the medications they took but because of the self-healing that took place in the body due to the intake of Dr. Sebi's alkaline diet.

Dr. Sebi's Nutritional Food Lists

Dr. Sebi's nutritional food lists are listed below:

Vegetable Diets
Izote flower and leaf, Kale, Mushrooms except for Shitake, Bell Pepper, Chayote, Cherry and Plum Tomato, Dulse, Garbanzo Beans, Arame, Wild Arugula, Avocado, Cucumber, Dandelion Greens, Amaranth, Watercress, Tomatillo, Turnip Greens, Wakame, Lettuce, Olives, Purslane Verdolaga, Squash, Okra, Hijiki, Nopales, Nori, Zucchini and Onions.

Fruit Diets
Peaches, Orange, Soft Jelly Coconuts, Cantaloupe, Prickly Pear, Cherries, Prunes, Bananas, Dates, Figs, Plums, Grapes, Apples, Pears, Limes, Mango, Berries, Raisins, Papayas, Melons, and Currants.

Alkaline Grains Diets
Kamut, Tef, Wild Rice, Spelt, Fonio, Amaranth, Quinoa, and Rye.

Alkaline Sugar Items

- Date Sugar.

- Agave Syrup from cactus (100% Pure).

Herbs Item

Dill, Onion powder, Basil, Pure sea salt, Oregano, and Cayenne.

Spices and Seasoning Diets

Dill, Achiote, Habanero, Savory, Basil, Thyme, Pure Sea Salt, Bay Leaf, Cayenne, Sweet Basil, Cloves, Onion Powder, Sage, Oregano, Powdered Granulated Seaweed, and Tarragon.

Herbal Tea Items

Elderberry, Tila, Burdock, Ginger, Fennel, Red Raspberry, Chamomile

CHAPTER 19

Benefits fo Dr. Sebi Treatments

D r. Sebi's Diet offers a lot of benefits to the dieters. While the foods recommended from this diet are known to reduce inflammation, there are other benefits that you can reap from following the Dr. Sebi Diet.

May Help with Weight Loss

While this diet regimen is not designed for weight loss, it can help people who want to lose weight. Studies show that people who consume an unlimited whole plant-based diet experience significant weight loss compa. How people lose weight with this diet relies on the high fiber and low-calorie foods that you are encouraged to eat. Except for avocadoes, nuts, seeds, and oil, most foods encouraged by the Dr. Sebi Diet are low in calories. But even if you consume nuts and seeds, they are not only calorie-dense but also rich in fiber and minerals.

Better Colon Health

Because this diet regimen encourages the consumption of large volumes of fruits and vegetables, it also has benefits to colon health. Foods rich in fiber can help promote healthy digestion; thus, people who follow the Dr. Sebi Diet do not suffer from constipation.

Appetite Control

Although many people think that this diet is very restrictive in terms of the amount of calories a particular person takes in, there are studies indicating that this diet can help with appetite control. The high fiber in your food can provide a high satiety level and can make one feel full for much longer.

Better Gut Microbiome

The stomach is the second brain. The enzymes and molecules released by the microbes in the gut affect not only your health but even your everyday mood. What you put inside your system also affects the kinds of molecules that the microbes release into the bloodstream. The type of food that you also consume can also affect the kind of microbes in your stomach. For instance, studies show that consumption of greasy, fatty, and processed foods can lead to the decline of good microorganisms and promote the growth of bad bacteria in the body.

Reduced Inflammation

While inflammation is one of the body's first line of defense indicating the presence of infection and diseases, chronic low-dose inflammation can also be bad to the body. In fact, the presence of chronic inflammation can result in many kinds of diseases such as diabetes, stroke, and even cancer. Thus, diets that are rich in fruits and vegetables are linked to reduced inflammation caused by oxidative stress. Studies that look into individuals consuming plant-based foods have a 31% lower incidence for developing heart diseases and cancer compared to those who consume animal products.

He created this diet for anybody who wants to prevent or cure any disease naturally. It can also improve your overall health without using chemical medications.

Dr. Sebi's theory is that all diseases are caused because of too much mucus building up in a specific area of the body. When you have too much mucus in your lungs, you get pneumonia. If you have too much mucus in your pancreas, it causes diabetes. He believes that any disease won't be able to exist in an environment that is alkaline but can happen if your body is too acidic.

Many people claim that his diet improved their health by using his compounds, and the herbal approach to heal the body worked better than any medical approach ever did. You can find many of his thoughts about herbal therapy and nutritional compounds on YouTube that help promote and teach healthy living long after his death.

His diet does offer many health benefits. The main one is it can promote weight loss because it restricts processed foods, and you will be eating more plant-based, unprocessed meals. This diet is full of whole fruits and vegetables that are full of plant compounds, minerals, vitamins, and fiber.

Diets that contains fruits and vegetables are related with oxidative stress and reduced inflammation, along with protecting you against most diseases.

Meatless diets have been linked to lower risks of heart disease and obesity. It also encourages foods that are high in fiber and low in calories. Regularly consuming fruits and vegetables can help protect your body against diseases and reduce inflammation.

If you can switch from your normal diet that is full of fast foods, saturated fats, refined sugars and grains to Dr. Sebi's diet could actually help you lose some weight—increasing your intake of grains, vegetables, and fruits while getting rid of pork and beef can decrease your risk of elevated cholesterol, high blood pressure, Type 2 diabetes, heart disease, and cancer. Most people eat way too much sodium, and this diet can drastically reduce lower this amount. This, in turn, can help you lower your blood pressure, and this reduces your risk of heart disease and stroke. In one study, people who ate seven servings of fruits and vegetables each day had between a 25 and 31 percent lower chance of heart disease and cancer.

Most Americans don't eat enough produce. During 2017 it was reported that between 9.3 and 12.2 percent met all their recommended daily intake of fruits and vegetables.

Dr. Sebi's diet encourages eating healthy fats like plant oils, seeds, and nuts along with whole grain that is rich in fiber. These foods have a lower risk of developing heart disease.

Any diet that limits processed foods can help you have a better quality of diet.

CHAPTER 20

Dr. Sebi STD Treatments

STDs, which stands for sexually transmitted diseases, are still fairly prevalent even though there are well-known ways to prevent them. There are numerous diseases that fall into the category of STDs and are spread by sexual intercourse, but can be spread through other manners. The most common STDs are trichomoniasis, syphilis, some types of hepatitis, gonorrhea, genital warts, genital herpes, Chlamydia, and HIV.

At one time, STDs were referred to as venereal diseases. They are some of the most common contagious infections. About 65 million Americans have been diagnosed with an incurable STD. Every year, 20 million new cases occur, and about half of these are in people aged 15 to 24. All of these can have long-term implications. These are serious illnesses that need to be treated. Some of them are considered incurable and can be deadly, such as HIV. Learning more about these diseases can provide you with knowledge on how to protect yourself.

STDs can be spread through oral, vaginal, and anal sex. Trichomoniasis is able to be contracted through contact with a moist or damp object, like toilet seats, wet clothing, or towels, although it is mostly spread through sexual contact. People who are at a higher risk of STDs include:

- Those who have more than one sexual partner.

- Those who trade sex for drugs or money.

- Those who share needles for drug use.

- Those who don't use condoms during sex.

- Those who have sex with a person who has had several partners.

Herpes and HIV are the two STDs that are chronic conditions that modern medicine can cure, but can only manage. Hepatitis B can sometimes become chronic. Unfortunately, you sometimes don't find out that you have an STD until it has damaged your reproductive organs, heart, vision, or other organs. STDs can also weaken the immune system, which leaves you vulnerable to contracting other diseases. Chlamydia and gonorrhea can cause pelvic inflammatory disease, and this can leave women unable to conceive. It is also able to kill you. If an STD is passed onto a newborn, the baby could face permanent damage, or it could kill them.

Causes of STDs

In terms of modern medicine, STDs are caused by all types of infection. Syphilis, gonorrhea, and Chlamydia are bacteria. Hepatitis B, genital warts, genital herpes, and HIV are all viral. Parasites cause trichomoniasis.

The STD germs live within vaginal secretions, blood semen, and, in some cases, saliva.The majority of the organisms will be spread through oral, anal, or vaginal sex, but some, like with genital warts and genital herpes, can be spread simply through skin-to-skin contact. Hepatitis B is able to be spread through sharing personal items, like razors or toothbrushes.

Prevention

The most obvious step in healing for STDs is to not get one in the first place. The first tip people give in preventing STDs is to not have sex, or at least avoid sex with people who have genital discharge, rash, sores, or other symptoms. The only time you should have unprotected sex is if you and your partner are only having sex with one another, and you have both tests negative for STDs in the last six months. Otherwise, you need to make sure you:

- Use condoms whenever you have sex. If you need a lubricant, make sure that it is one that is water-based. Condoms should be used for the entire act of sex. Keep in mind; condoms aren't 100% effective when it comes to preventing pregnancy or disease. However, they are very effective if you use them the right way.

- Avoid sharing underclothing or towels.

- Bathe after and before you have sex.

- If you are okay with vaccination, you can get vaccines for a lot of STDs, specifically Hep B and HPV.

- Make sure you are tested for HIV.

- If you abuse alcohol or drugs, please seek help. It is more common for people who are under the influence to have unsafe sex.

- Lastly, abstaining from sex completely is the only 100% effective way to prevent STDs.

There was a believe that using a condom with nonoxynol-9 would prevent STDs by killing the organisms that caused them. There are new study that has found that this can end up irritating the woman's cervix and vagina and could increase her risk of an STD. It is recommended that you avoid condoms with nonoxynol-9.

CHAPTER 21

Herpes Cure

An alkaline-rich diet that is rich in essential nutrients will help to rid your body of the herpes virus. This is achievable by creating an environment that can't support the growth of diseases causing substances.

The cells in the body needs oxygen to perform to their optimum capacity, but the chemicals and substances found in some medicines and foods rob your cells the much-needed oxygen to thrive.

Curing the herpes virus requires adequate cleansing of your body, and Dr. Sebi's plant-based alkaline diet does just that.

It is essential to know that curing herpes depends on the types of food eat and what you feed your body with.

You should avoid eating sweets and starchy foods. Eat foods that are bitter instead of sweet.

Eat more healthy vegetables such as zucchini, mushrooms, squash, cactus leaf or cactus plant flowers, and sea vegetables. Plant-based iron such as dandelion, burdock, yellow dock is also very helpful.

Dr. Sebi also emphasizes you practice fasting, because fasting helps you to eat less and heal fast. Another good reason why Dr. Sebi diet can cure herpes is that it gets rid of mucus in your body. This is because once your mucus membrane is compromised, your immune system becomes weak, and you become to disease.

Your mucus membrane needs to remain healthy for you to be healthy because it is your mucus membrane that is in charge of protecting the cells in your body.

The plant-based diets and herbs that are the main constituents of Dr. Sebi's alkaline cell foods are very effective for curing herpes.

Dr. Sebi was able to cure herpes by detoxifying the body and effectively nourishing the body.

The following steps were what Dr. Sebi used to cure herpes:
- Put an end to consuming acid foods. Ensure your body is not fed with acidic foods.
- Clean your body of acids and toxin, and start eating alkaline diets and herbs that increase the level of oxygen in your cells.
- Feeding your body with the needed nutrients that can repair, rebuild, and completely strengthen your body at the cellular level.
- Practice fasting. Take herbs and water only during fasting. You can add green juice if the fasting becomes too difficult for you.
- Eat vegetables and fruits immediately after fasting.
- Endeavor to eat foods from Dr. Sebi's nutritional guide after your body has been cured of herpes.

Detoxification is at the core of removing the body of the herpes virus-there is no other way that will bring the necessary results."

Some Facts about Dr. Sebi Diet for Herpes Cure
Dr. Sebi Diet herpes cure is anchored on some facts. Lets check some facts that made Dr. Sebi's diet for herpes cure so effective.
The Dr. Sebi diet is a plant-based alkaline diet is designed to eradicate acidity from the body and is effective in purifying and detoxifying the body.
Dr. Sebi's diet helps to strengthen the immune system and prime the body to fight off diseases such as herpes virus.
Dr. Sebi's diet helps to eliminate mucus, heal an already compromised mucus membrane, and empowers your body to heal itself of diseases such as herpes.

The Dr. Sebi Diet Products for Herpes
Dr. Sebi developed five effective herbal products that have helped a lot of people to heal herpes. These natural products are what you need to cure herpes.
Below are the main ingredients contained in Dr. Sebi's products for herpes.
- AHP Zinc Powder

- Triphala

- Pure extract giloy tablets

- Punarnavadi Mandoor

- AHP Silver Powder

Let us do a detailed analysis of the elements contained in these products.

1. AHP ZINC POWDER

The term AHP stands for ayurvedically herbo purified. The purification of zinc is done with decoctions of natural herbs such as Aloe Vera to produce AHP zinc powder.

AHP zinc power is of a better benefit than the usual zinc tablets you consume. AHP zinc powder is prepared from naturally occurring zinc, and that is what makes it very easy for your body to absorb.

AHP zinc powder also has the main qualities of some of the herbs used in preparing it. Modern medicine also acknowledges the importance of zinc for herpes treatment, but it is better to use AHP zinc powder instead of zinc tablets.

AHP zinc powder is safer and more effective in treating herpes.

2. Triphala

Triphala contains three outstanding herbal combinations. The three herbs that makeup Triphala are harad, amla, baheda.

These three herbs have not only been acknowledged for their potency by Dr. Sebi, but other medical experts have conducted research on these three outstanding herbs and praised its efficacy.

This herbal combination is a good combination that can be taken by both healthy persons and people that have the herpes virus.

This herbal combination can clean the unwanted materials and toxins in your body, and also help to purify your blood and many organs in your body.

Dr. Sebi didn't only administer this herbal combination to his patients, but he took daily for optimal health and longevity.

3. Pure Extract Giloy Tablets

Pure extract giloy tablets are produced manually from the extracts of the best quality Giloy. The Giloy used to make these tablets is gotten from the best quality Giloy.

Giloy is the perfect herb to improve your immunity and fight sexually transmitted diseases (STDs)

Dr. Sebi himself was a big fan of Giloy, and now, modern medical experts have accepted that Giloy can help your body to fight off many diseases and also helps in improving health.

4.   Punarnavadi Mandoor

Punarnavadi mandoor is not a herbs purified mineral, but a healthy herbomineral that is created from the combination of herbs and mineral.

Punarnavadi mandoor is an extraordinary combination of healthy minerals such as calcium, iron, and great herbs such as shunti, punarnava, alma, etc.

This herbomineral combination works perfectly on the liver and helps to eliminate toxins in the liver.

Dr. Sebi administered this herbomineral combination to many of his patients, and the reason for this is that the function of the liver was disrupted during infection, and Punarnavadi Mandoor is the perfect option to bring the liver function back to normal.

5.   AHP Silver Powder

Ayurvedically herbo purified (AHP) is a process that involves purifying various minerals in herbal decoctions making them useful for medication,

AHP ensures that the minerals do not only maintain their excellent abilities but absorbs the nutrition and qualities from the herbs, which they are purified into.

AHP powder is exceptionally helpful to your health, especially your nervous system. Dr. Sebi administered AHP silver powder to several of his patients with herpes, and the results were always good.

What makes AHP silver powder effective for herpes is that it works on your neurons. The very place where the herpes virus in your body use as their home and hiding place.

AHP silver powder works by sending the nanoparticles of silver into your neurons to eliminate and flush out the herpes virus in your neurons.

Curing Herpes with Dr. Sebi Diet on a Budget

The Dr. Sebi way of curing herpes is a simple process, and that is to nourish and detoxify the body. With this procedure, if you want to get rid of herpes on your body on a budget, here are some of the things you need to do:

1.   Herbs and fasting

The first things you can do is to fast during the detoxification period where you are taking in the necessary herbs alongside iron. On many occasions, Dr. Sebi has highlighted the importance of iron with regard to healing. This means that during this period, we can make use of the combination of green juices, water, and herbs for proper detoxification.

2.   Herbs and the Alkaline diet

Following the Alkaline diet while following the herpes healing process is important. The alkaline diet is one where you consume vegetables and other essential meals with the restriction of meat and other starchy meals.

The ingestion of starch and meat is something Dr. Sebi has stressed as something we need to avoid when healing herpes. We also have a recipe list that you can follow to help you stay on the Alkaline diet while curing your herpes.

This means that your body is cleansed of whatever might be fighting the healing process while you replenish the body and boost your immune system alongside.

Overall guide

At this point, you would avoid cooked food as much as possible.

You would also take out any acid-forming foods from your diet.

Fast while you take water and herbs.

Once you have completed your fast, you would need to take fruits and vegetables as they improve the healing process.

Once your herpes is gone, you would need to continue with the Dr. Sebi recipes for a while to keep you healthy and make the healing process a permanent one.

Herpes is curable as we know with all we have learned from Dr. Sebi, and it can be done on a budget as well. You do not need to spend a fortune to get this done, and all you have to do is follow the simple process highlighted here.

For Dr. Sebi herbs for herpes to work effectively for you, you have to start with the cleansing herbs.

Below are some of the cleansing herbs you need to take:

1. **Mullein**

   Mullein helps to cleanse the lung and also helps to activate lymph circulation in your neck and chest.

2. **Sarsaparilla Root**

   Sarsaparilla root helps to purify the blood and target herpes. Jamaican sarsaparilla roots are highly recommended because it is a great source of iron, and it is good for healing.

3. **Dandelion**

   Dandelion helps to cleanse the gallbladder and the kidney.

4. **Chaparral**

   Chaparral helps to cleanse harmful heavy metals from your gallbladder and blood and also cleanse the lymphatic system.

5. **Eucalyptus**

   You can use Eucalyptus to cleanse your skin through sauna or steam.

6. **Guaco Herb**

   Guaco heals wounds, cleanses the blood, promotes perspiration, increases urination, keeps your respiratory system healthy, and improves digestion. The leaves of Guaco can be used to relieve pain, treat some types of venereal disease, expel phlegm, reduce inflammation, thin the blood, and kill bacteria. You have to drink a lot of water when using the Guaco herb.

7. **Cilantro.**

   Cilantro helps to remove heavy and harmful metals from your cells, and this is essential for the healing of herpes because the herpes virus hides behind your cell walls.

8. **Burdock Root**

   Burdock root helps to cleanse the lymphatic system and the liver.

9. **Elderberry**

Elderberry helps to remove mucus from the lungs and upper respiratory system.

CHAPTER 22

Dr. Sebi Herbs for Herpes Cure

Dandelion

Dandelion herb is a root herb that is extremely rich in a chemical that helps to cure genital herpes. The sap of the dandelion is externally applied in a bid to reduce the proliferation of viruses into the cells. The sap can be gotten from either the root or stem of the dandelion. The extracted sap is to be rubbed on the genitals on a daily basis for an extensive period of 2 weeks. When this treatment is religiously followed, herpes symptoms would only last for a few more days.

Following the sap, the application routine is key to ridding your body of herpes symptoms. Unlike the medicinal cure, using this treatment for herpes have no side effects, no matter how long you use it.

Basil

Of all the discovered anti-viral herbs for herpes, this is simply one of the best. With its adaptogen, microbial, antioxidant, immune-modulating, and analgesic properties, basil leaves works like a magical cure for herpes. Basil is a popular ingredient for some other type of drugs, but its effect in helping to rid the body of herpes virus is lesser-known. Basil leaves, and its miraculous properties have greatly helped people with allergies. To get it right with the natural herpes remedy, you will need a batch of fresh basil leaves. These leaves are to be boiled in a cup of water for a few minutes, after which you can drink the resulting liquid once it cools down. This liquid herb is also an excellent alternative to tea. This mixture can be taken on a daily basis even when you do not have a herpes outbreak. However, during a herpes outbreak, ensure that you take this herbal drink twice a day. Taking this drink as much as you want on any given day will have no adverse effect on your body.

Lavender oil

Lavender essential oil, with its antiseptic and regenerative properties, is well known as a great natural cure for herpes. You can purchase a small bottle of lavender oil off the shelf of any supermarket. Unlike every other type of oil used in curing herpes, lavender oil has an inviting fragrance that will do well to compete with your cologne. A cotton swab can be used to apply the oil externally on cold sores two to three times a day. To avoid the infection propagating at other sites, ensure that you wash your hands thoroughly before and after applying the oil.

To make this natural herpes cure more effective, you can include jojoba oil with it to form a mixture. To further strengthen the effect, peppermint oil should also be considered in the mixture. These three essential oils in a mixture have been proven to be the most effective remedy to cure herpes. The extra-ordinary properties contained in the mixture of these oils will hasten the effect of the oils. After a proper mixture has been formed, a cotton ball can be dipped into it for a gentle but effective rub around cold sores. After rubbing the essential oils coated cotton swab around the cold sores, wash the sore area with cold water, afterward, dry the area with a dry cotton swab. During the herpes outbreak, the essential oil mixtures can be applied to the needed areas twice a day.

Olive leaf extract

Olive Leaf Extract for herpes treatment has been very effective. In the early 80s, to lower fevers and malaria effects, olive leaves were crushed and used in drinks for patients. In Moroccan medicine history, to stabilize blood sugar and control diabetes, olives were also used. During all these years of early usage, there was no regulatory body for the use of these leaves, and they worked wonders regardless. Now, in the scrutiny of learned medical professionals, several medicinal tests carried out on the olive leaves produced positive results all the way. Olive leaves have proved to be a unique and promising with several application methods. Now that olive leaves potency has escalated to scientific levels, now is your chance to try out olive leaves extract to cure your herpes with no hesitation and side effects.

How olive leaf extract eliminate herpes virus

Olive leaf extracts contain properties that are capable of removing viruses like HSV-1 and 2 with an inclusion of the Herpes Zoster virus. The potent property listed in olive leaves extracts is none other than the Oleuropein compound. This component is everywhere in an olive plant, from the trunk to the leaves. The compound happens to be away the plant protects itself from parasites. Lack of protein and stress has been found to be the main cause of a herpes outbreak. Basically, when your immune system weakens, the herpes virus rises. What the olive leaf extract does in the body is to give a boost to the immune system in a bid to prevent the herpes virus from breaking out. When ingested into the body, the olive leaf extracts tracks and attack the pathogens inside the body. During natural detoxification, the dead pathogens in the body are gotten rid of. The less toxin the body has, the lesser the likelihood of viruses and bacteria causing flare-ups.

Why Dr. Sebi Herpes Cure Is Your Best Option

By now, you already know what Dr. Sebi's herpes cure is all about. The reason behind this method of healing gaining grounds is not because a dime is being spent on an advertisement; instead, it is because of the way its effectiveness has captivated herpes patients. The effectiveness of De. Sebi's methods and principles have made him the talk of the town and a celebrated hero among herpes sufferers. We are going to use this medium to tell you why Dr. Sebi's herpes cure is the best option every herpes patient should go for.

Dr. Sebi was renowned as a herbalist who healed several patients who had already lost hope of getting any help. The herbalist simply identified the healing magic of herbs to make several individuals with incurable diseases free of an indemnity. When the same principle was applied to herpes, the result was unprecedented as well as unexpected. What the scientists have been unable to cure for ages, Dr. Sebi has been able to put them all under control. Until Dr. Sebi came into the picture, there was virtually nothing working on cold sores and other symptoms of herpes. This miraculous cure for herpes will give every herpes patient another chance at life. Knowing how to use Dr. Sebi's cure is important; what's more important is understanding why this traditional treatment is the best alternative around. Once this part is done and dusted, we will head straight into what this cure for herpes is made up of.

Why Dr. Sebi Cure for Herpes is the Best

It is best because it works in herpes: This is the best treatment so far from the effectiveness point of view. There is very little effective herpes treatment around the globe. There are antiviral drugs that are expensive yet ineffective. They only give a fake feeling of wellness when, in fact, nothing is working as it should in your body. Despite the intake of antiviral drugs by some herpes patients, the herpes simplex virus still thrives without any limitation. It is a lot of sacrifices to choose antiviral drugs over traditional medicines as the former only pamper the symptoms of herpes with a lot of underlying side effects. There are some other herbs that are safe but do not produce the same effect as Dr. Sebi's cure. This makes Dr. Sebi's cure the only solution that is perfect for every herpes patient as nothing comes close to its healing prowess.

It is the best option because it is the only safe option: Dr. Sebi's cure is all-natural, and all the ingredients contained therein are devoid of any synthetic material. Herbs have been in existence since the time the very first man was made, and the reason why they are still preferred over conventional medicine is the fact that they have zero side effects. Since Dr. Sebi's cure is entirely made up of herbs, you do not have to worry about your present and future health. As a matter of fact, these herbs work like magic, not only in curing you of herpes but also in improving your health every day. Those who have used Dr. Sebi herpes cure in the past have backed up the claim that these herbs indeed improved their health as they felt more energetic after starting the course. This makes Dr. Sebi herpes cure the only alternative you should consider.

- **It is best because it is cost-effective too:** With antiviral drugs, you need a prescription, Dr. Sebi herpes cure is different as you do not need prescription of any sort when you make a purchase. This alternative medicine tells you a lot of your money that goes into consultation. Health is important, but the money being spent on antiviral drugs is exorbitant, but that does not guarantee their effectiveness. On the other hand, Dr. Sebi's herpes cure is available on naturalherpescure.org. You do not need to pay a consultation fee, and zero marketing cost is involved. You only pay for what you get. Since this drug is effective and gets the job done, you are not throwing away your hard-earned cash.

- **It is best because it is certified by scientists:** Dr. Sebi's claim to cure herpes with herbs has been verified to be authentic by various medical and scientific researches. Some of the studies established more facts as to the antiviral properties of the herbs used in the herpes cure. Natural antiviral properties are able to rid the body of the herpes virus without any side effects. In addition to the antiviral properties found in these herbs, they have also been found to be immune-modulatory. This means they directly boost the body's disease-fighting mechanism. A stronger immune system simply means that the replication of the herpes simplex virus can be put under control in order for every herpes patient to live a herpes free life. All the researches about Dr. Sebi herpes cure approve it as the best solution for herpes.

- **It is best because it gives you herpes free life:** The efficacy of Dr. Sebi herpes cure is the sole reason why it is considered as the best herpes treatment all over the world. No other treatment has been verified to cure herpes, only this one can. You need to trust Dr. Sebi's methods so as to live a herpes free life.

The highlighted points are some of the reasons why Dr. Sebi herpes cure is the best one around. If you think it is time to put an end to the pains herpes is putting you through, you should give this cure a try. Before that, you must know the content of this cure. First and foremost is Giloy. Giloy came into limelight for its antipyretic properties, which match what is found in every antibiotic in the market. Years later, scientists realized that this herb relieves pain and enhances immunity

CHAPTER 23

Phlegm and Mucus

Phlegm is nothing more than a jelly-like mucus produced by the mucous membranes and these fluids are also expelled from the body through the lungs, bronchioles, and diaphragm. This waste is absolutely disgusting and disgusting. Getting in contact with phlegm makes you want to vomit. Phlegm doesn't have a definite perspective; sometimes it can be as clear as water; other times, it can be yellowish, green, dark, gray, light, or brown, depending on the type of food you eat. Some feel that the color of the phlegm expelled from your body is an indication of how healthy you are, but there is no substantial evidence to support this yet.

Phlegm can be compared to a chameleon that will take on the color of its surroundings. In this case, the color of the food consumed is considered. Mucus and phlegm are similar to inexperienced eyes, but they have their differences: one is more dangerous to human health than the other. You will soon find out how it happened.

What is mucus?

Mucus is basically a gelatinous liquid secreted by the mucous membranes; the consistency is thick and slippery. This liquid contains abundant water and glycoproteins.

Difference between phlegm and mucus

Mucus and phlegm are not identical, although most people consider them one. Let me explain, mucus is produced by our natural body as a defense mechanism. For example, mucus captures bacteria so they do not enter the body. But if you eat too many unnatural foods that cause your body to produce excessive mucus, that will be a problem, because your cells and organs will be starved of oxygen.

Phlegm brings disease

On the other hand, phlegm is very difficult to expel from the body. The presence of phlegm in the body is an indication that there is a disease lurking somewhere in the body. When phlegm is excreted in the body, mucus accompanies it, just like bacteria. This is yet another reason that phlegm is more troublesome for the body.

The relationship between food and disease.

Mucus disease

It is ideal to know the concept of disease, the environments in which it develops and the causes. This is the key to staying away from illnesses and ailments that your doctor will never tell you about. When we know these things, there will be no need for a healer, because getting sick will be rare.

Mucus is the cause of all diseases - Dr. Sebi

The disease is found in the body when you ingested a substance that does not live up to our body. This substance will conflict with our genetic structure and this will end up making us sick and weakened. Almost everyone usually gets sick because of the excess mucus in the body. The cause of most diseases is the presence of excessive mucus in the body.

When mucus accumulates excessively in the body, the mucous membrane breaks and the cells are covered with excess mucus. Basically, the mucous membrane serves to protect the body from invasion by aerobic bacteria.

Mucus and phlegm cause disease

When our diet consists of acidic foods, the mucous membrane breaks down and the mucus already secreted enters the bloodstream. When this happens, the other groups of cells that belong to the organs are deprived of oxygen. If the mucus reaches the nostrils, it is called sinusitis; when it flows into the bronchial tube, it is called bronchitis, and when it enters the lungs, it is called pneumonia. If mucus gets in your eyes, there will be a vision problem.

There you have it, three different diseases caused by mucus. There are more diseases; in the long list of other diseases caused by the invasion of mucus in various organs of the body are:

• Prostatitis ~ when mucus enters the prostate
• Endometriosis ~ when mucus enters a woman's uterus (this can cause yeast infections and vaginal discharge).

When you have symptoms of one of these diseases, the underlying cause is overproduction of mucus caused by an inadequate diet.

Phlegm after eating

Humans experience phlegm every time. When you cough with phlegm after eating, it is the result of consuming acidic foods. Now you understand that the overly acidic food you eat is the cause of your phlegm cough. If, after eating a certain type of food, you start producing a lot of phlegm through coughing, you need to stay away from that food. The production of excess phlegm due to the consumption of a certain type of food is an indication that that food is not healthy. Excessive secretion of phlegm will deprive your body of oxygen and other parts of your internal organs.

Symptoms of constant mucus in the throat.

Acidic foods do not complete the biological structure of the human body. The body's reaction to this is to make more mucus each time you eat acidic foods. The excess mucus in the lengths will spread to the throat. This situation will lead you to cough up phlegm after every meal you eat. A temporary solution to this condition is to gargle with salt water, but what is needed is a change in diet to prevent the body from producing excess mucus. If you refuse to change your diet to one that eliminates excess phlegm production, there will be more to cough up each time you eat acidic foods. Every organ in the body that houses this excessive mucus will experience one disease or another.

Herbs to relieve mucus and phlegm.

To help your body create a balance in mucus and phlegm production, herbs such as wild cherry bark, echinacea, slippery elm bark, chickweed, ginkgo biloba, burdock, and lobelia should be considered a essential part of your diet.

Mucus-free diet and mucus relief

- Avoid eating the following to help your body make excessive phlegm and mucus:
- White flour and white sugar are highly processed acidic foods that increase mucus and phlegm.
- Phlegm after eating eggs is due to excess mucus it creates in the body; it is difficult for the body to bring down a fetus, which is what eggs are.
- Phlegm after eating sugar is for the highly processed, artificial sweetener to break down and protect itself.
- Phlegm after eating bread is due to processed, dairy, and acidic ingredients like white flour, eggs, white sugar, or GMO grains. • Phlegm after eating dairy is due to thick phlegm and excess mucus that dairy produces in the body.
- Stop smoking and remove tobacco from your home Phlegm and mucus should not be played with, as leaving them unattended can lead to conditions such as pneumonia, lung congestion, acute bronchitis, chronic bronchitis, and bronchiectasis.

This featured guide should be followed carefully to remove excess mucus and phlegm in the body, as producing these two in excess eventually leads to disease.

CHAPTER 24

Dr. Sebi HIV Treatments

The same strategies to prevent any other STD are the same strategies that you should use to decrease your risk of contracting HIV. There are some medications that people can take that can keep them from contracting HIV, but these are normally only given to patients who are at a higher risk of contracting it.

Dr. Sebi offers an alternative to modern medicine when it comes to treating HIV. He believes that cleaning the mucus build-up in the lymphatic system and blood can help HIV.

Dr. Sebi didn't create something specifically to treat HIV/AIDS or any specific disease. Instead, he came up with compounds that are meant to cleanse the body and provide important nutrition. However, when you want to focus on cleansing your body of major illnesses, the interest will then turn to compounds that are found in his therapeutic packages.

We are all dealing with the fatigue and cellular stress because we are constantly exhausting out oxygen supply. And we are constantly trying to find any means to remain hydrated to deal with our suffocation through animal products, medical-chemicals, starch, and sugar.

We need out mucous membrane to maintain health because it helps to protect the cells. If this mucus is broken down, it becomes pus and will then expose your cells, which is what causes disease.

Now, when we are fasting, it will cause our bodies to form more oxygen. Then we start to provide our bodies with foods that are rich in potassium phosphate and iron fluorine, which helps to flush out toxins, tumors, and mucus from our internal walls. The reason we need to cleanse ourselves is that we know that our liver, intestines, and pancreas are power players for the best circulation. This will help to treat HIV/AIDS.

The only thing that is going to cause your body to start harming your mucous membranes is acid. This erosion in the body will create a greater oxygen deprivation. It is important that when you eat, you consume natural greens and fruits. Any grains you eat should not be man-made, and that all oils you use can retain nutrition once it is processed. Springwater will also help you to maintain your mineral content.

Dr. Sebi has come up with more than 40 herbs to flush your body of inflammation as well as nourish it. While many people will travel to Usha Village in Honduras to be cured of HIV/AIDs, you don't have to travel that far. All you need to do is stick to the nutritional guide and make sure you consume only alkaline foods.

The lymphatic system, skin, and blood make up the immunological system. It is important that you adhere to a strict diet to clear these areas of mucus. If you don't, it will take a lot longer to heal. To help boost your healing, you should consume only green leafy plants such as:

- Nori

- Hijiki

- Arame

- Dulce

- Wakame

- Burdock plants

- Lams quarters

- Purslane

- Nopales

- Dandelion greens

- Lettuce

You can also eat mushrooms, spices, and peppers that are on the approved foods list. When you start to follow this diet, it is important that you make sure you drink a gallon of water every day and do some light exercise. Having a gallon jug prepared for the day, at the start of the day, is a good idea, and you can count any water used in teas. You should drink red clover tea instead of chamomile.

The first thing you need to do is to address your iron deficiency because your immune system requires plenty of it. You need to take a bottle a day of either Bio Ferro or Iron Plus for ten days. After that, you only have to take two to three spoonfuls once you begin your therapeutic package. You can also consume a cup of bromide tea at noon and in the evening each day.

After that, the initial first ten days, you should start taking a mixture of different supplements. Some people will take all of them, while others only choose a select few. There are people on Dr. Sebi's website that can help guide you as to what you need to take. The following products are the ones you should look at:

- Electra Cell – breaks down calcification and strengthens your immune system, and clears out the build-up of mucus.

- Cell Cleanser – Gets rid of mucus, acids, and toxins on the intracellular level, and will improve your bowel movements.

- CC4 – Gets rid of mucus, acids, and toxins on a deeper intracellular level and will help provide you with mineral nourishment.

- Chelation – Helps to cleanse you on an intracellular level, and improves your bowel movements. It also helps your digestive tract.

- DBT –Helps to nourish and cleanse your pancreas.

- ECAL – Removes fluid and toxins from your cells' mitochondria. It is high in carbonates, phosphates, bromides, and iodides.

- Fucus – This is a natural diuretic. It will flush out stagnant fluids, dead cells, and promotes healthy skin. It contains phosphates, calcium, magnesium, and other important minerals.

- Lino – Get rids of calcification in the body. It has a lot of important minerals, which is important for the body and helps to break up and dissolve calcification.

- Lupulo – Calms the nervous system, relieves pain, and breaks up inflammation.

If you follow Dr. Sebi's diet and start taking his supplements, you can improve HIV/AIDs. That being said, it is still a good idea to continue to go to your doctor for monitoring. It is okay to take medications that your doctor prescribes while doing this. As you will read in the nutritional guide, the important thing is to take your supplements an hour before you take medications. This allows the supplements to help your body and heal your body from any ill-effects the medications could cause. Lastly, you may have noticed that Dr. Sebi's treatments for herpes and HIV are very similar. While there are slight differences, most treatments will follow along the same lines as these. That means if you start following the treatment for one disease, you will be helping to prevent other diseases.

CHAPTER 25

Revitalizing Herbs That Can Heal The Herpes Virus

R evitalizing herbs are herbs and oils that target the herpes virus specifically. It is important you take these revitalizing herbs after cleansing and detoxifying your body so that the herbs can completely clean your body.

Below are the Dr. Sebi Herbs that can heal the herpes virus

1. **Pao Pereira**

   Pao Pereira effectively helps to subdue the herpes virus, and it also inhibits the duplication of the herpes virus genome. This herb is an awesome herb to help to fight the herpes virus.

2. **Pau d'Arco**

   The chemical constituents contained in Pau d'Arco have shown in vitro anti-viral properties against HSV-1 and HSV-2, and other viruses such as poliovirus, influenza, and vesicular stomatitis virus.

3. **Oregano Essential Oil**

   Oregano essential oil is a great anti-viral that can suppress the herpes virus. It works best at ninety percent concentration. Apply essential oregano oil to your lower spine because your lower spine is the point where HSV-2 is dormant. You can also apply it to your genital area and under your tongue.

4. **Ginger Essential Oil**

   The ginger essential oil can kill the herpes virus on contact. But you should dilute the ginger essential oil with a carrier oil be used. The ginger essential oil has the same effect as oregano essential oil.

5. **Sea Salt Bath**

   Sea salt helps to absorb electrolysis through your skin and reliefs your skin during a herpes virus outbreak. To achieve this, you need to add a cup or half a cup of sea salt into a tub filled with warm water and soak your skin in it for some time. Ensure that the sea salt dissolves completely.

6. **Holy Basil**

   Stress is one of the factors that can trigger a herpes outbreak through adrenal fatigue. Holy basil is an adaptogen that relieves adrenal fatigue and prevents the outbreak of herpes through stress.

How To Extract Essential Oils For Herpes

There are numerous oils for herpes, and the one thing that we have to take into consideration is the extraction process.

The proper extraction of these oils from their natural sources is a delicate process which requires a lot of experience as well as the right materials.

There are numerous methods of extracting essential oils, but we are going to cover the two most important techniques, which are:

- **Steam distillation**
- **Cold Press**
- **Steam distillation**

The process of steam distillation makes use of steam and pressure for the extraction process. This process is a simple one, but without the right expertise, it can definitely go wrong.

The raw materials are placed inside a cooking chamber made of stainless steel, and when the material is steamed, it is broken down, removing the volatile materials behind.

When the steam is freed from the plant, it moves up the chamber in gaseous form through the connecting pipe, which goes into the condenser.

Once the condenser is cool, the gas goes back into liquid form, and this is the essential oil that can be collected from the surface of the water.

Cold Pressing

The cold press process extracts oils from the rind of the citrus as well as the seeds oil the carrier oil. This process requires heat but not as much heat as the steam distillation process with a maximum temperature of 120F for the process to go as planned.

The material which is heated is placed in a container where it is punctured by a device which rotates with thorns. Once the process of puncturing is complete, the essential oils are released into a container below the puncturing region. These machines then make use of centrifugal force to separate the essential oil from the juice.

Both processes are essential, and it has to be done properly with the right level of information from experts who know a lot about the process if not a lot of harm than good can and will be done.

CHAPTER 26

Detoxification of the Liver

In The Morning

You can start your morning with a cup of two or three mixture of any of the cleansing herbs tea/infusion. Take a brisk walk or bike riding or yoga or swimming.

After the exercise, your breakfast should be smoothie made with either: A handful of any of the veggies like kale, lettuce, Wild Arugula, Amaranth greens or asparagus (just one of the vegetable), 1 cantaloupe, ½ or 1banana (smallest and burros) and ¼ cup hemp or hazelnut milk.

You can try any of the green vegetables with, 1banana (smallest and burros), 2-3 key limes and 2-5 dates or any of the green mention above, ½ orange Seville, one green core apple, ½ cup of green grapes and 3-5 dates or any of the green vegetables, 16-ounce soursop pulp, 1/2 cup of papaya or 1 mango and 1 soft jelly coconuts or any of the green vegetable, 1head of elderberry, 1 core apple and 1 banana rip (smallest and burros).

Or any of your chosen veggies, ¼ to ½ peeled avocado (make sure the seed is removed), a cup of fresh fig and ¼ or ½ key lime or any of your choice green, 1 ripe cherimoya sugar apple, 1-2 ripe banana (smallest and burros), ½ or 1 key lime, 1 orange seville (optional) and Brazil nut or hazelnut milk.

Or Get a cup of zucchini, 1 or 2 mangos, 2 key lime, 1 orange seville and 2/3 to 1 cup of hazelnut or brazil nut milk or any of your choice green, 1 cup of hazelnut or brazil milk, 1 cup of fresh cherries and ½ cup of berries.
Take a Glass Of Spring Water After Every 2-3 Hours

In the Afternoon

Depending on the types of smoothies that you took in the morning, you can snack on watermelon, papaya, mangoes, apple, plum, pears, cherries, and other fruits that are in Dr. Sebi nutritional guide. (Please make sure what you are snacking on is not part of the recipes you used in making your morning smoothie.)

After snacking, take a cup of two or three mixture of any of the cleansing herbs tea/infusion.

In the Evening

You can eat delicious lettuce with tomato (plum and cherry), avocados, cucumber, olive oil, key lime, and drink a cup of two or three mixture of any of the cleansing herbs tea/infusion.

You can actually achieve any of the two types of cleansing by planning the other days like this.

How Long Do I Need To Detox My Body System?

The period of time that you need to detox your body system depends on your body's level of toxicity and tolerance level. However, late Dr. Sebi did 90-day detox, and he recommends 1-3 months as the best way to detox, but if you can't achieve that, you can do the 7-14 days detox. If you are sick or finding it difficult to fast on water, you can still fast on fruit and raw veggies from late Dr. Sebi's nutritional guide. Don't worry about the water or smoothies, and raw veggies fast as a result will come. The only difference is that the healing is faster, with the water fasting to the smoothies and raw veggies.

How Do I Prepare The Cleansing Herbs Infusion Or Tea?

For the making of the cleansing herbs infusion or tea, you can do that by using 1teaspoon of the herbs to 8ounce of water, and if you order a prepackage herbs, follow the dosage on the package herbs. However, to minimize the amount of water you drink per day, you can combine up to 3 different herbs together. That is one teaspoon each of the three different herbs to 8ounce of water.

Please make sure you don't combine more than 3herbs to keep the concentration at a good level. To combine herbs, ensure you do it in these ways: mix the gall bladder and colon cleansing herbs or kidney and liver cleansing herbs or mucus and respiratory cleansing herbs or heavy metal and lymphatic cleansing herbs.

Please note that, if you are on medication and you want to do a detox, you will have to take your medication an hour after taking your herbs and the colon herbs should not be consumed for more than 30 days so that your body system wouldn't have to depend on the herbs. Finally, reduce the dosage to 1 time per day or ½ teaspoon 2-3 times per day for the last three days of your fast.

To make the cleansing herbs infusion/tea using leaves or powder:
- Boil 8ounce of water (for one-time consumption)
- Measure one teaspoon of any of your cleansing herbs and if you want to combine herbs, measure one teaspoon each of the 2 or 3 different herbs and put it on your teacup/mug
- Pour the boiling water over the herbs and allow it to steep for 15-20 minutes.

Please note that herbal tea or infusion is the best way to consume the cleansing and revitalizing herbs as this is what late Dr. Sebi recommended at Usha village.

To make the cleansing herbs infusion/tea using root or extract:
a. Get your chopped root or extract and boil it for 15-20 minutes.

b. Allow it to get cold for 10-15 minutes.

CHAPTER 27

Dr. Sebi Diabetes Treatments

There isn't just one type of diabetes that a person can be diagnosed with. There are actually several different types. The most common forms are type 1, type 2, and gestational.

Type 1 diabetes is something that can't be avoided and is normally found in childhood, and is often referred to as juvenile diabetes. It is a type of auto-immune disease. In this case, your body doesn't make enough insulin. The immune system will also attack and destroy the pancreatic cells that create insulin. Most people with type 1 diabetes will have to take insulin every single day.

About five percent of people with diabetes have type 1 diabetes. Type 1 diabetes is considered incurable, but there are a lot of management tools out there. Some of the most common symptoms of type 1 diabetes are:

- Weight loss without an apparent reason

- Fatigue and tiredness

- Unclear or blurred vision and problems with sight

- Frequent urination

- Increased thirst and hunger

Once a person is diagnosed with type 1 diabetes, they enter the honeymoon phase. During this time, the cells that are responsible for secreting insulin could continue to make the hormone for a bit before stopping altogether. At this stage, they won't need as many insulin shots to keep their glucose levels.

This often causes the sufferer to think they are getting better. Even if things seem good, they need to make sure they are still closely monitoring their numbers. People with type 1 diabetes that go unmanaged can face dangerous complications. This can include:

- Diabetic retinopathy – Too much glucose can weaken the walls in the retina, which is the part of the eye that detects color and light. As this continues to progress, small blood vessels behind the eye could bulge and rupture, creating vision problems.

- Diabetic neuropathy – Too much glucose can reduce your circulation and damage the nerves in the feet and hands, which can cause pain, tingling, and burning sensations.

- Kidney disease – Since the kidneys filter glucose out of the blood, having to do this too much can cause kidney failure.

Some other issues people could face are depression, gum disease, and cardiovascular disease. Diabetic ketoacidosis is a complication that happens when the body is not given the right amount of insulin, and it places the body under great stress. This causes very high levels of blood sugar. At this point, the body has started to break down fat and not sugar and produces ketones. These ketones can become harmful if too many are produced, which causes acidosis. This is a medical emergency, and it will require hospitalization.

People with type 1 diabetes are faced with having to take insulin for the rest of their life. You will work with your doctor to figure out the best schedule for your insulin doses. There are now continuous blood sugar monitors and insulin pumps. This hybrid machine can act as artificial pancreas and remove the need for remembering when to take insulin. They will still need to manually check their blood sugar levels to make sure things are still okay.

Most of the time, for a person to develop type 1 diabetes, people are going to have to inherit a risk factor from both of their parents. It is believed that these factors tend to be higher in Caucasians because there is a higher rate of type 1 diabetes among Caucasians.
Since most people at risk for this don't develop diabetes, researchers want to figure out the environmental triggers. One trigger could be cold weather. Type 1 diabetes tends to show up more often during the winter months than summer and tends to be more prevalent in colder climates. They also believe that viruses could be another trigger. It is possible that a virus that has little to no effect on most can end up triggering type 1 diabetes in others.

Diet as an infant may also play a role. Type 1 diabetes isn't as common in those who breastfed and in those who started eating solid foods at a later age. For most people, developing type 1 diabetes tends to take several years.

A man with type 1 diabetes has a 1 in 17 chance of having a child who develops it as well. A woman with type 2 diabetes, and gives birth before the age of 25, there is a 1 in 25 risk that your child will develop it. If you give birth after the age of 25, the odds go down to 1 in 100.

A child's risk becomes doubled if you ended up developing diabetes before you were 11. If you and your partner have type 1 diabetes, the risk becomes 1 in 10 and 1 in 4. There are tests that can be given to find out your child's risk of developing type 1 diabetes.

Type 2 diabetes is acquired during life because of poor dietary choices, and sometimes genetics. It is most often caused by depleting your insulin resources to the point when the body is not able to make or use insulin correctly. This can be developed at any age, and even as a child. However, it is more common for middle-aged and older adults to be diagnosed. This is the most common form of diabetes. There are many risk factors for developing type 2 diabetes.

They can include:
- Leading a sedentary life
- Being older than 45
- Being of Asian-Pacific Islander, Latin American, Native American, or African American descent
- A History of PCOS
- Give birth to a child that weighed more than nine pounds, or having gestational diabetes
- History of high blood pressure
- Having an HDL cholesterol level that is less than 40 or 50 mg/dL
- Family history of diabetes
- Being overweight

The family lineage factor for type 2 diabetes is a lot stronger than it is for type 1 diabetes. Studies in twins have found that genetics plays a very big role in developing type 2. Yet, the environment still plays a big role as well. Lifestyle tends to play a very big role as well. Obesity often runs in families, and families will often have similar exercise and eating habits.

Gestational diabetes only affects women during pregnancy. For the most part, diabetes will go away once the woman gives birth, but it puts the baby at a higher risk of developing diabetes. The mother is also at a higher risk of developing type 2 diabetes later in life.

There are also less common types of diabetes, such as monogenic diabetes that is inherited, and diabetes-related to cystic fibrosis. As mentioned earlier, people can be diagnosed with pre-diabetes. Doctors diagnose people with pre-diabetes when blood sugar reaches a range of 100 to 125 mg/dL. Normal blood sugar levels are normally 70 to 99 mg/dL. A person who has diabetes will have a blood sugar high than 126 mg/dL when fasted.

Pre-diabetes simply means that you have a blood sugar level that is higher than it should be but isn't high enough to be considered diabetes. It does place you at a greater risk of developing type 2 diabetes. If a doctor finds that a person has pre-diabetes, they will suggest that the person start making healthy life changes to stop the progression. Eating healthier foods and losing weight will often prevent the development of diabetes.

While there is a lot of good advice for diabetics that doctors will share, such as lifestyle changes, there is also a lot of medication that you could end up being prescribed. And let's not get started on how scary it must be to learn how to give yourself insulin injections.

Dr. Sebi's diabetes cure is a super simple plan, and it doesn't cost that much. Very few people wanted to try his plan at first because it required fasting. Most would rather cut off their feet than not eat. Dr. Sebi was able to cure his diabetes with a 27 day fast.

There are a lot of other people who have reported similar results as well. You can find a lot of videos on YouTube, where people talk about having cured their diabetes with Dr. Sebi's plan. Like with the STD treatments, the goal is to rid the body of excess mucus. For diabetics, the excess mucus is found in the pancreatic duct. Dr. Sebi's own mother started fasting to help her diabetes, and after 57 days, she was cured.

During your fast, you should drink water, and you can also have herbal tea. A great herbal tea to drink is a combination of burdock, black walnut leaf, red raspberry, and elderberry. Use a tablespoon of each and mix them into one and a half liters of spring water. Bring this to a boil and let it steep for 15 minutes. Take this off the heat and mix in another half liter of water. Strain out the herbs and place to the side to use the next day. Store the tea in the fridge and drink as much as you want during the day.

A lot of people, when they hear the word fast, assume that means they can't take anything by mouth. But that's not Dr. Sebi's fast. See, when Dr. Sebi fasted to cure his diabetes, he would take three green plus tablets each day and drink sea moss tea, spring water, and tamarind juice. You don't have to drink tamarind juice, though. Any juice that is on the approved list of foods is okay. It must be fresh juice, though. You don't want pre-made juice with a bunch of added sugars.

Once you have fasted for a while, and your body will let you know when you have had enough, you will then need to start the Dr. Sebi approved diet plan. Along with that, you should also think about taking black seeds, mulberry leaves, and fig leaves. Research on black seeds has found that taking as little as two teaspoons of the powder each day can reverse diabetes.

Figleaves are the top alternative medicine for diabetes on the market today. Mulberry leaves are a common treatment for diabetes in the Middle East. These can be made into a tea, and you can mix in some black seeds as well.

Some other foods that you should consider adding to your diet are ginseng, okra, ginger, fenugreek, red clover, swiss chard, avocado, and bitter melon.

CHAPTER 28

Overcoming Hair Loss with Dr. Sebi

Hair loss is a problem that affects both men and women frequently, and it is accumulating over the years. Hair loss is most common in men as they experience complete baldness. However, women also experience hair loss through hair thinning, weakness, breakage, and falling off.

The following are Dr. Sebi's recommended herbs for hair growth and hair abnormalities treatment:

Marshmallow root: It is rich in proteins and vitamins. It helps in the treatment of hair problems such as eczema, psoriasis, and dry scalp, and it does this with the mucilage, which is a gel-like substance that becomes slippery when wet. It also helps in softening hair and helps in improving healthy hair growth. This herb could be also responsible for calming dry hair.

Nettle: It helps in alleviating hair loss through the stimulation of the scalp, improves blood circulation, and protects against further damage and breakage of the hair.

Licorice: It helps in moisturizing the scalp and hydrating the hair. This herb also prevents and fights many common hair problems such as dandruff, scabs, and itching. This herb can also be helpful in fighting baldness and improve hair growth.

Dandelion: This herb is rich in vitamin A, magnesium, iron, potassium, phosphorus, calcium, choline…and more. These nutrients are effective in improving hair growth through the treatment of the scalp and follicles.

Watercress: it is rich Vitamin A, biotin, and potassium. This makes it an excellent herb for the treatment of hair loss, helps active hair growth, nourishes the hair shaft, and supports the growth of fresh hair.

Flaxseed: it is rich in fatty acids that are essential for your hair and antioxidants that remove free radicals. It nourishes the hair, strengthens the hair, prevents hair loss, and soothes the hair.

Coconut oil: it helps in facilitating hair growth. Coconut oil is important in protecting the hair scalp and gives you smooth, shiny, and soft hair. This oil is also essential in preventing and fighting splitting and broken hair through strengthening the hair.

Sage: it contains antiseptic and astringent components that help in promoting longer, fuller, thicker, and shiny hair.

Preparation of the Herbs

- Rinse, dry, and grind the following herbs together dandelion, saw palmetto, sage, nettle, marshmallow, licorice, watercress, and flaxseed.

- Collect half tsp. of each herb and add into two cups of water.

- Boil for about five minutes.

- Drain and drink two times daily.

Note:

- You can collect half tsp. of each herb and boil with three cups of water.

- Steep and used to wash your hair once in a day.

Or:

- Collect two tbsp. of undiluted coconut oil and two tbs. of olive oil.

- Add two tbsp. of powdered thyme and curry herbs.

- Mix thoroughly and apply to your hair.

- You can add the mixture to your hair cream and apply it thoroughly.

Non-Dr. Sebi's Herbs for Hair Growth and Hair Problems

Some other herbs are effective for improving hair growth and fighting hair abnormalities. These herbs are regarded as non-Dr. Sebi's herbs.

These non-Dr. Sebi's herbs are:

Aloe Vera: the constant usage of this plant's gel on hair helps in sustaining the pH of the hair. It helps in making the scalp conditioned and also improves hair health. It facilitates the opening up of the obstructed pores in the scalp and increases the growth of hair follicles, thereby improving hair growth.

Sesame Oil: sesame oil is rich with vitamins, omega fatty acids, and all other nutrients necessary for hair growth and hair abnormalities. This oil is important for improving hair health through fighting hair problems such as ringworm, dandruff, head lice, dryness, psoriasis…and more. Sesame oil facilitates hair growth, prevents and fights hair abnormalities, prevents hair and scalp exposure from U.V light. Constant use of sesame oil may cause your hair to become dark; hence, this oil is beneficial for individuals growing gray hair.

Almond Oil: this oil is loaded with Vitamin A, and E. almond oil is very effective in fighting scalp infections and inflammation and many other hair problems.

- **How to Use Sesame Oil, Almond Oil, and Aloe Vera Gel**

This mixture is very effective for fighting the above-mentioned hair problems as well as improving hair growth.

- Collect about one tbsp. of sesame oil, almond oil, and add the same proportion of Aloe Vera gel.

- Place on a pan that is capable of heating the mixture.

- Allow the mixture to heat properly for about 2 minutes.

- Allow it to get cool slightly and apply on your scalp by thorough massaging.

- Allow it to stay on your hair for about 40 minutes.

- Rinse with shampoo.

Ginseng: this is another natural herb that helps in preventing and fighting hair loss. It increases the transfer of blood from the bloodstream to the scalp, thereby ensuring the hair follicles receive enough blood and nutrition, giving way for healthy and strong hair.

It is very effective in combating baldness and helps hair growth: hence, increasing fuller, longer and stronger hair.

Neem: Neem leave is very effective for improving hair and scalp health. This plant helps in increasing the easy supply of blood through the blood vessel to the scalp. When this happens, hair is expected to grow quickly thus, preventing hair loss and untimely hair gray.

Rosemary: have you heard about any herb that is capable of detoxifying the hair scalp? Rosemary is a special herb that can help you do that. Because when you detoxify your scalp, it helps you prevent hair loss and hair abnormalities. Rosemary helps in making your hair stronger, especially your hair root.

Amla (Indian Gooseberry): this herb is rich in vitamins C, B complex, iron, calcium…and more. It is used very widely for treating hair loss here in India. Amla does many functions for your hair when used regularly: it conditions and strengthens the hair and also promotes hair growth.

Chinese Hibiscus: this is a powerful herb that helps in preventing premature greying of the hair and it also promotes hair growth. Many hair problems are managed with the use of this herb.

Moringa: This plant is very effective in providing strength for the hair follicles and helps in preventing hair from falling out. Moringa is also used as a natural conditioner and facilitates hair growth.

Lavender oil: Lavender oil contains antibacterial, antimicrobial, antiseptic, and anti-inflammatory components. It is essential in fighting baldness, increasing hair growth, and improves hair health. His oil helps in fighting hair and scalp problems such as head lice, dandruff, dry scalp, and many other scalp infections. The constant use of this oil assists in preventing hair from falling off and facilitates rapid hair growth. You can use this oil by applying it on your scalp and hair and massage very well to ensure penetration of the oil on the hair.

Preparation

- Rinse, dry, and grind the following herbs Ginseng, Neem, Rosemary, Amla (Indian Gooseberry), Chinese Hibiscus, and Moringa separately.

- Collect a half tsp. of each herb and add into two cups of water.

- Boil for about five minutes.

- Drain and drink two times daily.

On the other hand,

- You can collect half tsp. of each herb and boil with three cups of water.

- Steep and used to wash your hair once in a day.

CHAPTER 29

Overcoming Lupus with Dr. Sebi

Lupus is a horrible long-term autoimmune disease where your body's own immune system gets hyperactive and begins to attack healthy, normal tissue. Some symptoms can include damage, swelling, and inflammation to your lungs, heart, blood, kidneys, skin, and joints.

Because of its complex nature, some people call lupus the "disease of 1,000 faces." There are, on average, about 16,000 new cases of lupus every year in the United States. There are over one million people who are living with lupus. Lupus normally only affect women and happens between age 15 and 44.

In 2015, lupus gained attention when Selena Gomez announced she was diagnosed in her teen years and had taken treatments for it. Lupus isn't contagious, and it can't be transmitted in any way to another person. There have been some extremely rare cases where a woman with lupus gave birth to a child who developed a type of lupus. This is known as neonatal lupus.

Types of Lupus
There are several types of lupus. The main ones are neonatal, drug-induced, discoid, and systemic lupus erythematosus.

Neonatal
Most of the babies who are born to mothers who have systemic lupus erythematosus are usually healthy. About one percent of all the women who have autoantibodies that are related to lupus will give birth to a child with neonatal lupus.
The mother might have no symptoms, Sjogren's syndrome, or SLE. Sjogren's syndrome is another condition that can happen with lupus. Most of the symptoms include dry mouth and dry eyes.

If a baby is born with neonatal lupus, they might have low blood count, liver problems, or a skin rash. About ten percent have anemia. The rash will normally go away within a couple of weeks. Some infants will have a congenital heart block. This is when the heart can't regulate a rhythmic and normal pumping action. The baby might need to have a pacemaker. This could be a condition that is life-threatening. If you have SLE and want to get pregnant, you need to talk with your doctor before and make sure they keep a close watch on you during your pregnancy.

Drug-induced

About ten percent of all the people who have SLE will have symptoms that show up due to a reaction to specific drugs. There are about 80 drugs that can cause this condition.

These could include some drugs that are used to treat high blood pressure and seizures. They might include some oral contraceptives, antifungals, antibiotics, and thyroid medicines.

Some drugs that are associated with this type of lupus are:

Isoniazid: this is an antibiotic that is used in the treatment for tuberculosis
Procainamide: this is a medicine that is used to treat heart arrhythmias.
Hydralazine: this is a medicine that is used to treat hypertension.
This type of lupus normally goes away once you stop taking the specific medication.

Subacute Cutaneous Lupus Erythematosus

This refers to lesions that appear on the skin that was exposed to the sun. These lessons won't cause any scarring.

Discoid Lupus Erythematosus

With this type of lupus, the symptoms only affect the skin. Rashes will appear on the scalp, neck, and face. These areas might become scaly and thick, and scarring might happen. This rash could last from a couple of days to many years. If it does go away, it might come back.

DLE doesn't affect any internal organs, but about ten percent of all the people who have DLE will also develop SLE. It isn't clear if the people already had SLE, and it only showed up on the skin or if it progressed from DLE.

Systemic Lupus Erythematosus

This is the most common type of lupus. This is a systemic condition, meaning that is can impact any part of the body. Symptoms could be anywhere from extremely mild to extremely severe.

This one is the most severe of all the types of lupus because it can affect any of the body's systems or organs. It could cause inflammation in the heart, blood, kidneys, lungs, joints, skin, or a combination of any of these.

This type of lupus normally goes through cycles. During remission times, the patient might not have any symptoms at all. When they have a flare-up, and the disease is very active, their symptoms will reappear.

Causes

We know that lupus is an autoimmune disease, but one exact cause hasn't been found.

What happens?

Lupus happens when our immune systems attack healthy body tissues. It is more than likely that lupus is the result of a combination of your environment and genetics.

If a person has an inherited predisposition, they might develop lupus if they come in contact with something in their environment that triggers lupus.

Our immune systems will protect our bodies and helps to fight off antigens like germs, bacteria, and viruses. This happens because it produces proteins that are called antibodies. The B lymphocytes or white blood cells are what produce these antibodies.

If you have an autoimmune condition like lupus, your immune system can't tell the difference between healthy tissue, antigens, or unwanted substances. Because of this, our immune system will direct the antibodies to attack the antigens and healthy tissues. This can cause tissue damage, pain, and swelling.

An antinuclear antibody is the most common type of autoantibody that develops in people who have lupus. These ANA react with the cell's nucleus. All these autoantibodies are circulated throughout the blood, but some of the cells in the body will have walls that are thin enough to allow some autoantibodies to move through them.

These autoantibodies could attack the body's DNA in the cells' nucleus. This is the reason why lupus will affect certain organs but not others.

Some possible triggers might include:

Medications: Lupus could be triggered by some blood pressure medicines, antibiotics, and anti-seizure medicines. People who get drug-induced lupus normally get better once they stop the medicine. Symptoms rarely persist after they stop the drug.

Infections: Getting an infection could cause a relapse or initiate lupus in certain people.

Sunlight: Being exposed to the sun could trigger an internal response or cause skin lesions in certain people.

Why the Immune System Goes Wrong?

There are some genetic factors that play a role in the development of SLE. Some of the genes in the body can help the immune system to function properly. People who have SLE, these changes could stop their immune system from working right.

One theory relates to the death of cells. This is a natural process that happens as the body renews cells. Some scientists think that because of some genetic factors, the body doesn't completely rid itself of all the dead cells. The cells that are dead and stay in the body might release substances that make the immune system malfunction.

Risk Factors

You might develop lupus due to many different factors. These could be environmental, genetic, hormonal, or any combination of these.

Environmental

Environmental agents like viruses or chemicals might contribute to causing lupus to show up in certain people who might be genetically susceptible.

Some possible environmental triggers could be:

Viral Infections:

These might trigger some symptoms in certain people who are susceptible to SLE.

Medications: About ten percent of most cases of lupus could be related to a certain drug.

Sunlight: Being exposed to sunlight can trigger lupus in some people.

Smoking: The rise in more cases in the past several decades might be because of being exposed to tobacco.

Genetics

Scientists haven't proved that one certain genetic factor can cause lupus, even though it is a lot more common in some families.

Genetics might be the cause of the following risk factors:

Family History

Anyone who has a first or second-degree relative who has lupus will have higher risks of getting lupus. Scientists have found specific genes that might contribute to getting lupus. There just hasn't been enough evidence to prove that they actually cause the disease.

In some studies, done with identical twins, one twin might get lupus while the other doesn't, even if they did grow up together and have been exposed to the same environmental factors. If one twin has lupus, the other one will have about a 25 percent chance of getting this disease, too. Identical twins are more genetically imposed to have this condition.

Lupus could happen to people who don't have any family history of this disease, but there might be other autoimmune diseases within the family. Some examples include idiopathic thrombocytopenic purpura, hemolytic anemia, and thyroiditis.

Some researchers think that changes to the X-chromosomes might increase the risk.

Race

People of a certain background can develop lupus, but it is about three times more common in people who have an African background as compared to Caucasians. It is also more prevalent in Native American, Asian, and Hispanic women.

Hormones

These are chemicals that get produced by the body. They help to regulate and control activities of certain organs or cells.

This hormonal activity might explain these risk factors:

Age

The diagnosis and symptoms usually happen between the ages of 15 and 45, basically, during a woman's childbearing years. But about 20 percent of all cases happen after a woman turns 50.

Since nine out of ten lupus diagnoses are female, scientists have looked at a link between lupus and estrogen. Women and men produce estrogen, but women do produce more.

In one study done in 2016, some scientists found that estrogen could affect the immune activity and cause lupus antibodies to develop in women who are more susceptible to lupus.

This could explain who autoimmune disease will affect more women than men. During 2010, scientists published a study that reported women who had been diagnosed with lupus reported more fatigue and pain when menstruating. This might suggest that symptoms might flare more during this time.

There just isn't enough evidence that will confirm that estrogen actually causes lupus. If there is an actual link, an estrogen-based treatment could regulate how severe lupus gets. A lot more research is needed before doctors will offer it as an actual treatment.

Gut Microbiota

Researchers have recently been looking at gut microbiota as one factor in developing lupus. Scientists say specific changes to gut microbiota happened in both mice and people who have lupus. They need more research in this area.

Can Children Be at Risk?

Lupus is very rare in children who are under 15 years of age if their birth mother didn't have it. If their birth mother had it, they might have lupus-related skin, liver, or heart problems.

Infants who have neonatal lupus might have higher chances of getting a different autoimmune disease later in their life.

Symptoms

During flare-ups is when people who have lupus will feel the symptoms. During times between the flare-ups, people won't have any or only a few symptoms.

Lupus has many symptoms, and these include:

- Arthritis
- Purple or pale toes or finger from stress or cold

- Unusual hair loss
- Chest pain when taking deep breaths
- Headaches
- Fever
- Sensitive to sun
- Mouth ulcers
- Skin rashes caused by bleeding under the skin
- Swollen lymph nodes or glands
- Swelling around the eyes or in the legs
- Swelling or pain in the muscles or joints
- Weight loss and a loss of appetite
- Fatigue

Systemic Lupus Erythematosus

This type of lupus can affect people in various ways, and symptoms can happen to different body parts, such as:

- Joints and Muscles
- Swollen joints
- Arthritisaches and pain
- Blood
- High blood pressure
- Anemia
- Heart
- Atherosclerosis
- Inflammation of the fibrous sac
- Endocarditis
- Skin
- Red or butterfly patches
- Stomach
- Severe pain
- Kidneys
- Blood in urine
- Lungs

CHAPTER 30

Diagnosis and Symptoms

Diagnosis
Getting a diagnosis can be hard since all the various symptoms might resemble the symptoms of other illnesses. It is also hard since the symptoms and signs will vary greatly for each person. The symptoms and signs might vary with time and overlap those of other illnesses.

There isn't one test that can diagnose lupus. Your doctor will ask you about symptoms, do an examination, and take a family and personal medical history. They will take into consideration the 11 criteria that I mentioned above. Your doctor might also request some blood testing along with other laboratory tests.

Image Tests
If you or your doctor thinks that your lupus is affecting your heart or lungs, they might suggest that you have either:

- Echocardiogram: This test utilizes sound waves to make images in real-time of your heart while it is beating. This checks for problems with the valves and other parts of the heart.

- Chest X-ray: This is an image of the chest that might reveal shadows that might an inflammation or fluid buildup in the lungs.

Other image tests could help your doctor to see any organs that are affected by lupus.

Tissue Biopsy
Your doctor might also request a biopsy. Lupus could harm the kidneys in several ways, and treatments vary depending on the kind of damage that happens.

There might be a time when it will be necessary for your doctor to take a sample of your kidney tissue to find out what treatment would be best. This sample gets taken through a small incision or with a needle. Skin biopsies are sometimes done to see if lupus is damaging your skin.

Urine Test

These can help your doctor diagnose and monitor the effects that lupus is having on your kidneys. They are looking for cellular casts, white blood cells, red blood cells, and protein that could help show how your kidneys are working. For some of these tests, just one sample is needed. For others, the person might have to collect several samples over a 24-hour time frame.

Blood Tests

This can show if specific biomarkers are present. These biomarkers can give your doctor information about which one of the autoimmune diseases you might have.

Erythrocyte Sedimentation Rate

This is a blood test that shows how fast red blood cells settle on the bottom of a tube in one hour. If they settle faster than normal, this might show lupus. This test isn't specific to just one disease. It could be elevated if you have cancer, other inflammatory conditions, an infection, or lupus.

Serum Complement Test

This measures how much protein your body consumes when inflammation occurs. If you have low levels, this shows that inflammation is present in your body and that your SLE is active.

Anti-histone Antibodies

These are proteins that have a role when creating DNA. People who have drug-induced lupus normally have them, and anyone who has SLE might have them. These won't necessarily confirm a diagnosis.

Anti-La/SSB and Anti-Ro/SSA Antibodies

There is about 30 to 40 percent of all the people who have lupus will have anti-La/SSB and anti-Ro/SSA antibodies. These can happen with people who have Sjorgren's syndrome and anyone who has lupus but tested negative for ANA.

They can be present in a tiny amount in around 15 percent of the people who don't have lupus, and it can happen with other conditions like rheumatoid arthritis. If a woman has anti-Ro and anti-La antibodies, there might be a chance that her baby will have neonatal lupus after birth. Anyone who has lupus and wants to get pregnant will need to be tested for these specific antibodies.

Anti-U1RNP Antibody
About 25 percent of all the people who have lupus will have anti-U1RNP antibodies. People who don't have lupus will have less than one percent of these antibodies. This antibody might be present in someone who has Jaccoud's arthropathy and Raynaud's phenomenon, which is a deformity of the hands caused by arthritis.

Anti-Smith Antibody
About 20 percent of all the people who have lupus will have an antibody to Sm, which is a ribonucleoprotein that will be present in the cell's nucleus. It will be present in less than one percent of all people who have lupus. It is extremely rare in people who have other rheumatic diseases. Because of this, anyone who has anti-sm antibodies will likely have lupus, too. It isn't normally present with kidney lupus.

Anti-dsDNA Antibody
This is the anti-double-stranded DNA antibody, which is a certain kind of ANA antibody that happens in about 30 percent of everyone who has lupus. Less than one percent of people who don't have lupus will have this type of antibody. If you test positive, it might mean that you have a serious form of lupus-like kidney lupus or lupus nephritis.

Anti-DNA Antibody Test
About 70 percent of all the people who have lupus will have an antibody called the anti-DNA antibody. This will normally cause a positive when you are having a flare-up.

Antiphospholipid Antibodies

APIs are kinds of antibodies that are directed against phospholipids. APIs will be present in about 50 percent of all the people who have lupus. People who don't have lupus could have APLs, too. Anyone who has APLs could have a higher risk of pulmonary hypertension, stroke, and blood clots. There is also more of a risk of complications during pregnancy, including miscarriage.

Antinuclear Antibodies

About 95 percent of all the people who have lupus will have positive results when taking the ANA test. Some people who test positive for ANA, but won't have lupus. Other tests will have to confirm this diagnosis.

Biomarkers

These are genetics, proteins, antibodies, and other factors that will show your doctor what is happening with your body or how your body is responding to treatments. These are useful because they could show that a person has a condition even if they don't have any symptoms. Lupus could affect different people in different ways. This makes it hard to find biomarkers that are reliable. But doing a combination of tests, including blood tests, could help your doctor determine your diagnosis.

Monitoring Tests

Your doctor will continue to do tests to find out how lupus is affecting your body and how well your body responds to treatments.

Home Remedies and Treatments

There isn't a cure for lupus, but the flares and symptoms can be managed by medication and lifestyle changes. The treatment that your doctor chooses depends on your symptoms and signs. Figuring out whether your symptoms need to be treated and with what medicines need to be carefully considered. Your doctor has to take into account all the risks and benefits.

As your symptoms and flares lessen, your doctor might decide to change your dosage or medicines.

These are the medicines that are normally used to control lupus:

- Rituximab

This is beneficial if you have a resistant strain of lupus. Some side effects might be an allergic reaction to the infusion, and an infection could happen.

- Biologics

This is a different kind of medicine. The most common is Benlysta, and it gets administered intravenously. It can reduce the symptoms in some people who have lupus. Some side effects are infections, diarrhea, and nausea. Sometimes depression might get worse.

- Immunosuppressants

These are drugs that suppress the immune system and might be helpful in the more serious cases of lupus. Some examples of this type of drug are Trexall, CellCept, Azasan, and Imuran. Some side effects might include the risk of cancer, decreased fertility, liver damage, and infections.

- Corticosteroids

Prednisone is the most popular type of corticosteroid. These drugs can help with the inflammation caused by lupus. High doses like Medrol or Methapred are used to control serious diseases that damage the brain and kidneys. Some side effects are infections, diabetes, high blood pressure, thinning of the bones, easy bruising, and weight gain. The risk of these side effects will increase with higher doses and longer therapy.

- Antimalarial Drugs

These medicines are normally used to treat malaria-like Plaquenil. These can affect the immune system and could help to decrease flares. Side effects could include damage to the retina and upsetting the stomach. Normal eye exams are recommended when you take these medicines.

- NSAIDs

Taking over the counter NSAIDs like Motrin, Advil, and Aleve can be used to treat fever, swelling, and pain associated with lupus. Stronger NSAIDs can be obtained by prescription. Some side effects include increased risk of developing heart problems, kidney problems, and possibly stomach bleeding.

Treatments try to:
- Reduce organ damage
- Manage or prevent flares

Medications could help:
- Control cholesterol
- Reduce infections
- Manage blood pressure
- Prevent or reduce organ and joint damage
- Balances hormones
- Regulates the immune system's activities
- Reduces swelling and pain

Your exact treatment depends on how lupus is affecting you. If you don't do any treatments, flares can happen that could have life-threatening consequences.

Lifestyle Changes

You need to take steps to take care of yourself if you have been diagnosed with lupus. There are simple measures that can help you prevent lupus flares, and if they do happen, help you cope with the symptoms you have experienced. You need to try to:
- Calcium and vitamin D Supplements

Talk to your doctor about these. There is evidence that suggests people who have lupus might benefit from taking a vitamin D supplement. A 1200 to 1500 mg calcium supplement might keep your bones healthier.
- Eating Healthy

A healthy diet will include whole grains, along with fresh vegetables and fruits. Your doctor might give you some dietary restrictions if you have gastrointestinal problems, kidney damage, or high blood pressure.

- Stop Smoking

Smoking can increase your risk of getting cardiovascular disease and could make the effects of lupus on your blood vessels and heart.

- Exercise

Make sure you exercise regularly. Exercise can keep your bones strong and helps to reduce the risk of having a heart attack. It can also promote a general well being.

- Sun Smart

Since ultraviolet light can cause a flare, you need to make sure you wear protective clothing like long pants, long-sleeved shirts, and a hat. Make sure you use sunscreen that has an SPF factor of no less than 55 each time you head outside.

- Visit Your Doctor

Make sure you have regular checkups rather than just seeing your doctor when your symptoms get worse. This could help your doctor prevent flares and could be useful when addressing routine concerns like exercise, diet, and stress. This can help prevent complications from lupus.

Alternative Medicine

Some people who have lupus look for complementary or alternative medicine. There aren't many alternative therapies that can change the course of lupus, even though some could help to ease the symptoms.

Talk about these treatments with your health care provider before you try them by yourself. They can help you weigh the risks and benefits and will be able to let you know if they will interfere with your current medicines. Some of the alternative and complementary treatments might include:

- Acupuncture: This treatment uses tiny needles that are inserted just under the skin. This could help ease the muscle pain that is associated with lupus.

- Dehydroepiandrosterone or DHEA: Try to find supplements that contain this hormone. It could help with muscle pain and fatigue. It could cause acne breakouts.

CHAPTER 31

The Cure of Cancer in Dr. Sebi Way

D r. Sebi's first step to the cure of cancer was cleansing and detoxification of the body while the second step is revitalizing the body. Sufferers are advised to stop eating foods that are not recommended in Dr. Sebi's food lists if they need to be cured in Dr. Sebi's way.

He recommended detoxification procedures that will remove any form of mucous and toxins in the body. This cleansing and detoxification process involves the employment of Dr. Sebi's herbs that contains strong detoxification agents.

His cleansing and detoxification process is quite holistic in the sense that it detoxified different organs such as Liver, Gall bladder, Kidney, Lymph glands…and many others. Hence, no matter the grade in which breast cancer has developed, the detoxification process will remove all the forms of toxins present in there.

All the intracellular and intercellular regions of the body will also be detoxified.

- **Dr. Sebi 21 Days Fasting To Cleanse and Detoxify the Body**

In order to achieve perfect cleansing and detoxification, you must adhere to the following strictly:

1. Drink one gallon of water every day.

2. Drink tamarind juice each day.

3. Constant exercise is needed.

4. You must not eat any food other than the ones prescribed in this book.

5. When you are done with the detoxification and cleansing process, you are not expected to go back to your formal habit of eating.

6. Learn to continue the intake of alkaline diets even after the completion of your treatment, as this will help you maintain your health and live a healthy life.

7. Ensure you take Irish Sea moss every day.

How To Prepare Irish Moss

- Use warm water to rinse out any attached dirt and debris found in the plant.

- Add 10 cups of clean water to two cupsful of Iris moss.

- Place in a source of heat with the use of a large cooking pot and cook for about 25-30 minutes.

- Allow it to become soft and form a paste.

- Add one cupful of water to it again and blend it until smooth.

- Then consume it every day.

The herbs Dr. Sebi used for cleansing and detoxification are:

- **Eucalyptus**: cleanses the skin with the use of the steaming process.

- **Rhubard root**: detoxifies the tone and digestive tract wellbeing.

- **Dandelion**: detoxifies the kidney and gall bladder.

- **Mullein**: detoxified the lung and activated the lymph circulation in the chest and neck.

- **Elderberry flower**: detoxifies the upper respiratory system by removing mucus from it, and it also detoxifies the lungs.

- **Chaparral**: detoxifies the lymphatic system and clears heavy metals from the blood and gall bladder.

- **Burdock root**: detoxifies the liver and the lymphatic system.

- **Cascara Sagrada**: It helps move stool through the bowels by causing muscle contractions in the intestine.

Preparation of the Herbs and Dosages

- Collect each of the herbs from a reliable source.

- Rinse them thoroughly with clean water.

- Expose them to direct sunlight to make them dry thoroughly.

- Grind each herb separately to powder form.

- Preserve them in a dry and clean container.

- Collect one tsp of each of the above plants and add three cups of alkaline water.

- Boil them for about 5 minutes.

- Remove from the heat source and leave it for a few minutes to get cool.

- Drain before consumption.

- Take one cup of the herb two times daily. This should be taken daily for 21 days.

After you have achieved your detoxification and cleansing, the next step is the use of herbs needed for the cure of breast cancer.

Let us proceed by describing and introducing the method of preparation of the herbs required for the complete cure with the accurate curate cure you have to take.

- **Herbs Used to cure Breast Cancer in Dr. Sebi's Way**

After the 21 days of complete fasting with herbs, water, and juice, Dr. Sebi proceeded in the cure of breast cancer. The herbs used for the cure of breast cancer are:

Sarsaparilla Root
This plant contains a high source of iron that is essential for healing cancer disease.

Anamu (Guinea Hen Weed)
This plant is very effective in fighting cancer cells.

Soursop
This plant is better than chemotherapy, and it fights against cancer. Several types of research had been carried on in this plant to observe its effect on the cancer cell.

In one study, they looked at the effect of this plant on leukemia cells, and it was found out that it stopped the growth of these cells. The extract of this plant was also used in a breast cancer cell, and it was observed that the extract was able to diminish the size of the tumor, kill the cancer cells, and made the body immuno-competent.

Pao Pereira

This plant is proven scientifically to kills cancer cells of the breast, ovary, brain, and pancreas. This herb is a great one. It is a tree from the amazon rain forest and is employed as an alternative medication to treat above-listed cancer.

During a research study, this plant's extract was applied to a culture, the extract supports the growth of cells, which in turn killed the cancer cells. Not only that, but it also caused a total reduction in the size of tumor cells. This means it contains tumor-suppressing activities and can also be utilized for the prevention of cancer disease. This plant attacks only the cancer cells and does not attack other cells as chemotherapy does.

Cannabidiol (CBD) oil with Tetrahydrocannabinol (THC)

It can also be used to cure cancer. Dr. Sebi used this plant in his village, but in most cases, he does prefer other plants mentioned above.

Preparation of the Herbs and Dosages

- Collect the herbs from a reliable source.
- Rinse them thoroughly with clean water.
- Expose them to direct sunlight to make them dry thoroughly.
- Grind each herb separately to powder form.
- Preserve them in a dry and clean container.
- Collect one tsp of each of the above plants and add three cups of alkaline water.
- Boil them for about 2-3 minutes.
- Remove from the heat source and leave it for a few minutes to get cool.
- Drain before consumption.

Take one cup of the herb three times daily until your result is obtained

CHAPTER 32

Dr. Sebi's Cure for Kidney Disease

B asically, any problem with your kidneys might lead to your blood not being purified well. This causes toxins to be accumulated in the blood. You might have a family history of kidney problems, high blood pressure, and diabetes. Recent studies show that overusing normal medications for various diseases can play a huge role in deteriorating the health of your kidneys.

Many people are habitual users of medications, even for the slightest aches and pains. You have probably done it since you didn't know that these drugs could harm your health, including your heart, liver, and kidneys. Many people today have moved to a more holistic approach for their health. Dr. Sebi knew what some scientists are trying to prove today. He might have known that people today would need his help in curing their kidney problems. Yes, he created a herbal remedy for kidney problems.

If you have been diagnosed with kidney disease, following Dr. Sebi's diet can help you. Make sure you talk with your doctor if you feel like something isn't quite right with your health. When you think about all the toxins being put into our bodies today, it isn't any wonder that there are so many people with kidney problems.

Ingredients in the Kidney Disease Kit

Dr. Sebi's kit combines many very healthy and rare herbs that he thought was perfect for any kidney problem. Unfortunately, not all problems can be treated with the same herbs. Dr. Sebi's kits let you customize them for your needs. Let's look at the ingredients:

- UTI Special Mix: UTIs are the most common problem with kidneys. If you are constantly getting UTIs, this might help you stop getting them.

- Kidney Stone Hunter: This herbal mix works against kidney stones. Even if you don't get kidney stones, this can help detoxify your body.

- AHP Zinc Powder: AHP or ayurvedically herb purified zinc powder can be taken by anyone who has a zinc deficiency. Zinc deficiency can cause kidney problems.

- Swarna Bang Tablets: This combination of herbs has been used for thousands of years to fight recurring UTIs. These are strong enough to help the kidneys, too.

- Chandanadi Tablets: This herbal combination includes Daruharidra-Berberis aristata, sandalwood oil, karpoora, rala-shorearobusta, amalaki, acacia catechu, kattha, gandhabirojasatva, sugandhamaricha, and sandalwood. These herbs are combined in the correct proportion to get the perfect outcome.

- Punarnava Special Kidney Mix: Some reports published about kidney disease claims panarnava is one herb that help the kidneys function properly.

Benefits

As you know, your kidneys are a critical filtration part of your body. Without it, we wouldn't be able to survive for long with all the toxins we are exposed to everyday. Even the slightest of imbalances in filtering out toxins, we could be faced with problems like cysts, kidney stones, UTIs, gout, or other chronic and severe complications. Some are fairly common, but others can be life-threatening.

Dr. Sebi's kidney kit gives your body the minerals and herbs your body needs to keep your kidneys healthy. They can help your body function better by detoxifying your body. The herbs help to cleanse the kidneys of all the toxins it has stored up. This won't happen overnight; it will take several months for you to notice any results. Each kit will last for about two months.

When you go to Dr. Sebi's website, there will be some questionnaires for you to feel out. These will help them pick the right combination of herbs for you. You will then get to decide what you want to try in order to improve your health.

CHAPTER 33

Dr. Sebi's Natural Cure for High Blood Pressure

What Are The Basis To Heal High Blood Pressure Naturally?
In other to heal high blood pressure naturally, there are things that you must do:

1) You must follow Dr. Sebi's alkaline plant-based diets.
2) Consume at least 1 gallon of spring water daily.
3) Consume an only a moderate amount of sea salt and avoid table salt completely.
4) Make sure you don't consume more of grain, including alkaline grain.
5) Ensure you are not suffering from any kidney or thyroid disorder that can trigger hypertension because if you are, then you have to address that first.
6) Change your diet: this is a must (maintain an alkaline diet) for you to treat high blood pressure.

What Are Dr. Sebi Steps To Healing From Hypertension?

Irrespective of the disease or sickness that you want to cure, there are certain processes that cannot be changed with Dr. Sebi methodology. The steps are cleansing or detoxification, revitalization, and dieting.

What Is Cleansing/Detoxification?

Cleansing or detoxification: this step has to do with an intra-cellular cleansing of your entire cells by eradicating mucus from your body system (intra-cellular cleansing) using Dr. Sebi approved fast, spring water green smoothies, and cleansing herbs.

What Is Revitalizing?

Because during the cleansing period and while suffering from the disease, your body will lose a lot of energy, so after cleansing/detoxification, you will need to regain all the energy that your body have lost by revitalizing your body system with the revitalizing herbs to strengthen your immune system and nourish and replenish the loss energy of your body system.

What Is Dieting?

These have to do with changing your eating habit: that is, eating only foods that are listed in Dr. Sebi's nutritional guide. Dr. Sebi state that a lot of people were not able to treat themselves of hypertension completely because they cannot change their diet system, but if you can follow Dr. Sebi's approve diet, you will certainly be free from high blood pressure.

Below are what to and not to eat in Dr. Sebi's nutritional guide.

The lists of vegetables recommended by Dr. Sebi are:

- Kale
- Bell Peppers
- Garbanzo Beans (chickpeas)
- Lettuce (no Iceberg)
- Mexican Squash (Chayote)
- Mexican Cactus (Nopales)
- Zucchini
- Okra
- Mushrooms
- Onions
- Asparagus
- Squash
- Amaranth Greens
- Wild Arugula
- Tomato (plum and cherry)

The lists of Fruits recommended by Dr. Sebi are:

- Grapes seeded
- Apple
- Bananas (smallest and burros)
- Chirimoya sugar apple
- Cherries
- Plums
- Figs
- Tamarind
- Limes and key limes w/seed
- Mangoes
- Prickly Pear
- Orange Seville or sour
- Cantaloupe
- Papaya
- Prunes
- Raisins (seeded)

- Berries
- Curants
- Pears
- Soursops
- Peaches
- dates
- Soft jelly coconuts
- Melons (seeded)

The list of nuts and seeds recommended by Dr. Sebi are:

- Walnuts
- Hazelnut
- Raw Sesame Seeds
- Brazil Nuts
- Hemp Seed

The lists of oil recommended by Dr. Sebi are:

- Olive oil
- Coconut oil
- Avocado Oil
- Grape seed Oil
- Hemp seed Oil

The list of spices and seasonings that Dr. Sebi recommended are:

- Pure Sea Salt
- Cayenne
- Thyme
- Basil
- Sage
- Onion Powder
- Cloves Dill
- Oregano
- Habanero

The lists of grain recommended by Dr. Sebi are:

- Kamut

- Wild rice
- Amaranth
- Quinoa

The lists of flour recommended by Dr. Sebi are:

- Quinoa flour
- Teff flour
- Rye flour

The lists of things that Dr. Sebi recommends that we should avoid are:

- All types of meat, including white and red meat.
- Dairy product like: eggs, milk, cheese, yogurt, butter etc.
- All types of sugar (including cube and powdery)
- Garlic
- All human-made food (can and package food)
- Do not use microwaves

What Are The Source Of Disease And How To Get Rid Of The Root Cause Of Hypertension?

Before talking about the sources of all types of disease, there is a need to define what disease is. So, what is disease? According to Oxford learners dictionaries, "disease is an illness affecting humans, animals or plants, often caused by infection" whereas, Dr. Sebi defines disease "as the compromising of the mucous membrane.

When I said the mucous membrane is compromised, I mean that the mucous membrane has been broken. So, wherever the mucous membrane got broken or compromise determines the sickness that will manifest.

He further states that there is only one disease, which is the mucus (inflammation)." Take it or leave it, there is only one disease, and the source to all the types of diseases is the mucus.

Below is a table showing you where the mucous membrane gets compromise and the sicknesses that will manifest:

S/No.	Point Of Membrane Compromised	Sickness
i.	Lungs	pneumonia, cystic fibrosis, (COPD) chronic obstructive pulmonary disease
ii.	bronchial tubes	Bronchitis
iii.	Trachea	Hemoptysis, wheezing and Stridor
iv.	Reproductive organ	Fibroid or low sperm count, infertility, endometriosis etc.
v.	Pancreatic duct	Diabetes
vi.	Retina of the eye	Blindness or blur sight
Vii	kidney	Kidney stone, acute kidney injury etc.
Viii.	Brain	Parkinson, paranoia, insomnia etc.
Ix	Joint	Arthritis
x	heart	Heart failure, high/low blood pressure etc.
And	A lot	More

This was the reason why Dr. Sebi, disagrees with the idea of cleansing only one part of the body, which is the colon, but believes in cleansing the entire body system. According to late Dr. Sebi, the only way to get rid of the root cause of hypertension is through an intra-cellular cleansing (cleansing/detoxification) of the whole cells because the whole body is interconnected and cleansing of one cell without the others is as good as not cleansing at all as the un-cleanse cells will infect the cleanse cells.

So, by undergoing an intra-cellular cleansing, means that you are resetting your entire cells from the Colon to the Lymph glands, Liver, Gallbladder, Kidney and the skin back to its original state (alkaline environment) where no disease will be able to withstand and revitalize the body system to recover from the energy that it has loosed due to the presence of the disease.

What Is Detox/Cleanse?

Detox Or cleanse is an alternative-medicine or treatment that helps in getting rid of toxins (mucus) that have been accumulated in the body system, which have either a short or long term effect on human health.

What Are The Various Types Of Detoxification Or Cleansing?

Although there are various types of detoxification I am going to center on fasting, which is the one approved by late Dr. Sebi.

Under the fasting method of detoxification, there are various types of fasting which include:

i. **Dry fasting:** Under this type of fasting, you will abstain from food, water, juice, anything eatable or drinkable.

ii. **Liquid fasting**: under this type of fasting, you are to abstain from anything solid and consume only liquid-like; juice and any other liquid stuff without alcohol.

iii. **Water fasting:** under this type of fasting, you are to abstain from anything solid, juice, smoothies, etc. and consume only water.

iv. **Fruit fasting:** under this type of fasting, you are to avoid anything solid but survive mainly on fruit.

v. **Raw food fasting**: under this type of fasting, you are to abstain completely from cooked food and survive mainly on veggies and fruit.

vi. **Smoothie fasting:** smoothie fasting is just like the fruit fasting; the only difference is the fact that under smoothie fasting, the fruit will be blended, and you will also consume blended veggies.

Bear in mind that Dr. Sebi approved 12 days fast with alkaline herbs, sea moss, spring water, and alkaline juice, which must be made with fruit that is in Dr. Sebi's nutritional guide list.

What Are The Step By Step Method On How To Do A Detox Or Cleanse (Intra-Cellular Cleansing)?

Are you ready to cleanse or detox your body system now? Let's get started. Depending on the types of fasting you will want to undergo, but I am recommending water fasting. Whichever type of fast that you decide to do, you will still need to consume the alkaline herb's tea/infusion daily.

However, when detoxifying or cleansing your body system, you will experience some symptoms like:

i. Sleeplessness

ii. Catching a cold or flu

iii. Rashes or itching and sometimes, pain and ache

iv.The tongue might be discolored

v. Your bowel movement will change

vi. Lack of energy (low energy)

vii. Your blood pressure might be low (rare symptoms)

viii. Possible breakouts

ix. Expel mucus

You don't have to worry yourself with these symptoms as it won't last up to a week, so don't get scared; it is the process of cleansing.

Furthermore, I will walk you on how to make a detox with water fast, green smoothie and raw veggies.

How To Do A Detox With Water Fast

In the morning: start up your morning with a cup of two or three mixture of any of the cleansing herbs tea/infusion. If possible, you can consume spring water before or after the cleansing herbs. Make sure you don't consume anything except water throughout the number of days that you want to fast.

In the afternoon: take a cup of two or three mixture of any of the cleansing herbs tea/infusion. You can equally take water. Please note that you are to be taking a glass of spring water every 2-3 hours.

In the evening: Take a brisk walk or bike riding or yoga or swimming. Once you are done with the exercise, take your cleansing herbs. You are good for the day. You can apply this system every other day for the number of days that you decide to observe the water fast.

For those of us who will find it difficult to undergo the water fast, you can try the green smoothies and raw veggie fast.

CHAPTER 34

Dr. Sebi Approved Cleansing Herbs For

Hypertension

There are a lot of cleansing herbs, but it depends on whether you are doing a general cleansing or cleansing for a particular disease. For Hypertension's cleansing, below are the cleansing herbs:

1.   Cascara Sagrada: this is a purgative and laxative herb that helps in cleansing of the colon, moves stool through the bowel, and stimulate liver and pancreas secretion.

2.   Rhubarb Root: is also a laxative that is effective in improving the health of the digestive tract and eliminating heavy metals and harmful bacterial from the body system.

3.   Prodigiosa: is a cleansing herb that is used for both cleansing and revitalization. It helps to cleanse the blood and gallbladder, dissolve kidney stones, stimulate pancreas secretion, and reduce blood sugar level.

4.   Burdock root: Burdock root is a cleansing herb that helps to cleanse/detox the liver and lymphatic system, eliminate toxins through the skin, purifies the bloodstream, boost sex drive (libido) and lower high blood pressure.

5.   Chaparral: this is another cleansing herb that aids in the cleansing of the lymph system, helps to shrink tumors, prolapsed uterus, venereal disease and kidney, and bladder disorder, and gets rid of heavy metals from the blood and treat diabetes.

6.   Dandelion: This is another herb for detoxification that is rich in calcium and helps to cleanse the gallbladder, kidney, and bloodstream and also dissolve kidney stones, relieve diabetes, liver, and urinary disorders.

7.   Elderberry: this is a cleansing herb that helps in eliminating mucus from the upper respiratory system and the lungs and also induce sweat and urine to purify the body system.

8.   Guaco: this is another cleaning herb that is rich in iron and potassium phosphate that helps to cleanse the blood system, eliminate mucus/phlegm, heals wound, increase the rate of urination, promote healthy respiration and perspiration, enhance digestion, treat venereal diseases, reduce inflammation, damage harmful bacteria, thin blood, relieve pain and a lot more.

9.   Eucalyptus: this cleansing herb, helps in cleansing the skin through steaming/sauna

10.   Mullein: mullein is also one of my favorite cleansing herbs that aids in the cleansing of the lungs and lymphatic system, remove mucus from the small intestine and also, helps in activating the lymph circulation in the neck and chest.

What Is Cascara Sagrada?

Cascara sagrada is a shrub plant from the family of Rhamnaceae. It is called different names in different languages. Some of it names include cascara, sacred bark, frangula purshiana, cascara buckthorn, rhamni purshianae cortex, California buckthorn, yellow bark, ecorce sacree, chittem stick, pastel bourd, bearberry, dogwood bark, nerprun, purshiana bark, Sagrada Bark, rhamnus purshiana, rhubarbe des paysans etc. this plant is a native to western North America from southern British Columbia. Most people are familiar with this plant as a "dietary supplement," and were saleable in the pharmacies as over the counter drugs (OTC). In the year 2002, FDA declares that the plant does not meet the standards or requirements to be sold as over the counter drugs (OTC). Before then, the dietary supplement or the bark of Cascara Sagrada has been used for centuries as a purgative for constipation and laxation that helps to cleanse the colon.

How Does Cascara Sagrada Works?

Because of the chemicals compound that Cascara Sagrada contained like: hydroxyanthracene glycosides, cascarosides-A, B, C, and D, emodin and anthracoid, research has it that it can help trigger peristalsis by preventing the absorption of electrolytes and water in the large intestine which in turn will lead to an increase in the volume of the bowel contents, that will now lead to increased pressure.

The hydroxyanthracene glycosides compound is hydrolyzed by intestinal flora to help form what is absorbable in the colon. So, whenever the cascarosides is hydrolyzed, it will form aloins, like; barbaloin and chrysaloin. The compound or substance that it contains that is known as; emodin also helps to make it serves as an effective laxative.

What Are the Benefits Of Using/Consuming Cascara Sagrada?
The benefits of using/consuming Cascara Sagrada include:
- It helps to serve as a laxative for constipation.
- It helps to cleanse the colon.
- It is used for the treatment of gallstones.
- It is used for the treatment of liver problems.
- It is used to treat cancer.
- It is used to treat digestive problems.
- It helps in relieving joint and muscle pain.
- It is used for the treatment of gonorrhea
- It aids in relieving gallstones
- It is used for the treatment of dysentery
- It is used as a bitter tonic.

What Are The Side Effects Of Cascara Sagrada?
Although there are no side effects recorded for consuming cascara sagrada in less than a week orally there are some possible side effects that one can suffer from if it is consumed constantly for more than a week. These possible side effects are:
- Stomach irritation or cramps
- Dehydration
- Heart issues
- Muscle weakness (please note that the last two side effects are very rare.)

What Are The Precaution To Beware Of Before Using/Consuming Cascara Sagrada?

The precaution to beware of before using Cascara Sagrada includes:

- Pregnant and breast-feeding mothers should not use cascara sagrada because it can induce labor on pregnant women, and for breastfeeding mothers, their baby might suffer diarrhea.
- Cascara sagrada is not good for children as they easily get dehydrated. This, in turn, will make the child lose a lot of electrolytes like potassium.
- Do not use these herbs for more than a week.

If you have a history or suffering from any of the diseases below, do not use this herb:

- Ulcerative colitis or Crohn's disease.
- Stomach discomfort or pain with an unknown cause.
- Any kind of kidney disease
- Intestinal Obstruction
- Irritable bowel syndrome
- Colitis
- Hemorrhoids

What Are The Medications That Interacts with Cascara Sagrada?

Cascara Sagrada interacts with certain drugs. These drugs include:

1. Digoxin (Lanoxin): since Cascara sagrada serves as a stimulant laxative that is very effective in decreasing potassium levels in the body, and digoxin does the same thing, combining the two medications together will lead to potassium deficiency from the body system

2. Any medication made for inflammation (Corticosteroids): since Cascara Sagrada has the potency to reduce potassium in the body and medication made for inflammation has the same potency, consuming both Cascara Sagrada and any medication for inflammation will certainly lead to potassium deficiency. Medication for inflammation includes:

- Water pills (Chlorothiazide)
- Furosemide (Lasix)
- Prednisone (Deltasone)

- d.Dexamethasone (Decadron)
- Methylprednisolone (Medrol)
- Chlorthalidone (Thalitone)
- Hydrocortisone (Cortef).

3. Stimulant laxatives interact with Cascara Sagrada: consuming two different stimulant laxatives will only lead to dehydration and low minerals in the body. Stimulant laxatives medications include
- Fletcher's Castoria
- Dulcolax
- Senna (Senokot)
- Castor oil (Purge)
- Correctol
- Bisacodyl (Dulcolax/Correctol)
- Black Draugh
- Senokot Senexon
- Feen~A Mint
- Carter's Little Pill

What Is The Dosage And How To Prepared Cascara Sagrada Tea/Infusion?

For the dosage and how to prepare cascara sagrada tea or infusion, kindly take the steps below:

1. Pour 1~3grams of your fine chopped bark of Cascara Sagrada in 8ounce of water.
2. Steams it for 10 to 15 minutes on your cooker
3. Once it is the stem, strain it to remove the chopped bark of cascara sagrada.
4. For the dosage, consume 1 to 3 grams if you are using the dried bark and if it is the powdered bark, consume 1 to 2.5 grams 2~3 times daily.

What Is Rhubarb Root?

Rhubarb Root is the underground stem. That is the rhizome of the Rhubarb plant. The root of this plant is called different names by different people. It names include Rhubarbe Palmee, Da Huang, Ruibarbo, Chinese Rhubarb, Rhubarbe Potagere, Turkey Rhubarb, Rheum tanguticum, Indian Rhubarb, Rheum Officinale, Himalayan Rhubarb, Rhubarbe Medicinale, Rhubarbe Indienne, Rheum emodi, etc. however, the root of rhubarb plant has been used for centuries by the traditional Chinese people for the treatment of various ailment.

How Does Rhubarb Root Work?

Because of the chemicals compound that Rhubarb root contains like; anthraquinones, emodin, rhein and stilbenoid like; rhaponticin and flavanol glucosides, catechin and fiber, research has it that, the root is a very effective laxative that has the potency to reduce pains from inflammation, treat swelling, cold sores and improves the health of the digestive tract, purifies the blood stream by clearing of heavy metal from the blood, eliminate harmful bacteria, reduce cholesterol levels and improve the general movement of the intestines.

What Are The Benefits Of Using/Consuming Rhubarb Root?

The benefits that you will enjoy from using or consuming Rhubarb Root are:

1. It is used to treat cold sores and herpes simplex virus.
2. It is used to treat canker sores.
3. It helps to enhance and improve the symptoms of menopause.
4. It helps to treat and prevent pancreatitis (swelling of the pancreas).
5. It helps to improve the respiratory system of people that are having or suffering from ARDS to breathe better and healthier.
6. It helps to relieve dysmenorrhea (menstrual cramps or pain).
7. It helps to treat bleeding in the stomach.
8. It is used to treat gastrointestinal (GI) bleeding.
9. It helps to lower cholesterol levels or body weight.

What Are The Side Effects Of Using Or Consuming Rhubarb Root?

Till at the time of writing this book, there are no side effects that anyone has ever recorded about consuming Rhubarb root and it rhizome for a period of 2 years but the consumption of it leaves orally is 100% unsafe because of the oxalic acid that the leaves contains.

What Are The Note-Full Precaution Of Using Or Consuming Rhubarb Root?

The note-full precautions before using/consuming this plant are:

1. Do not use this root if you are pregnant or breast-feeding mothers as consuming more than the amount in food can be detrimental.
2. It can worsen the situation for people that are suffering from diarrhea or constipation.
3. Do not use this root if you are suffering from kidney disease or kidney stones as it can harm the kidney and form kidney stones.
4. If you have any liver disorder, do not use rhubarb root as it can make the liver malfunction.

What Are The Medications That Interact With Rhubarb Roots?

Medications that interact with Rhubarb roots include:

1. Just like cascara sagrada, rhubarb root interacts with Digoxin (Lanoxin).
2. Any drugs that is made for inflammation (just like Cascara Sagrada)
3. Water pills and warfarin (Coumadin) interacts with rhubarb root.
4. Just like cascara sagrada, rhubarb root interacts with laxatives stimulant.
5. Medication that has the potency to harm the kidney interacts with Rhubarb, and they include:

   - Aminoglycosides; (amikacin/Amikin)
   - Ibuprofen (Nuprin/Motrin/Advil)
   - cyclosporine (Sandimmune/Neoral,)
   - Piroxicam (Feldene)
   - gentamicin (Gentak/Garamycin)
   - Naproxen (Anaprox/Naprelan/Aleve)
   - Indomethacin (Indocin)
   - Tobramycin (Nebcin) etc.

What Is Dosage And How To Prepared Rhubarb Root Tea/Infusion?

For the dosage and how to prepare Rhubarb root tea/infusion, kindly take the following steps:

1. Uproot the root of Rhubarb plant (ensure the plant is above four years and it is during autumn); you can order for the root online.
2. Wash the roots under running water to remove all dirt and remove the external fibers and dried it.
3. After drying it, chopped it into smaller pieces (less than 0.5 inches) or pound it and stored it in a tightly closed container.
4. Whether you order online or you have the pounded or chopped rhubarb root, you can prepare it by pouring 1tablespoon of the pounded or chopped rhubarb root in 1 cup of 8 ounces (240 ccs) of water to make a tea.
5. Boil the mixture for 15 minutes and reduced the heat of the gas for about 10 minutes.
6. Put off the fire and allow it to get cold for 15 minutes and strain the root.
7. For the dosage, take 8ounce of the infusion three times a day.

CHAPTER 35

Dr. Sebi Cleansing Herbs

What Is Prodigiosa?
Prodigiosa is also known as 'Prodijiosa, Amula, Hamula, Brickellia Grandiflora herb, Bricklebush, Brickellia, etc.' is a perennial plant with large bushy leaves and flowers and it's from the daisy family and native to Mexico and California. These plants have a grey-purple hue on the underside and dark green leaves on the upper side and can grow up to 5feet height with its flowers growing in clusters. This plant has a long history with the Mexicans as it has been used for centuries for the treatment of; diabetes, arthritis, diarrhea, and stomach disorder and relieve aching joints.

How Does Prodigiosa Work?
Because of the chemical and compound composition of Prodigiosa, research has it that it is very effective for the treatment of diabetes II because of how it aids in stimulating the pancreatic gland to secret and reduces or lowers blood sugar level and burn down fat in the gallbladder. The irony is that Prodigiosa can cause more damage to people that are suffering from Type I diabetes. Furthermore, consuming Prodigiosa's tea/infusion helps to boost the digestion of fat and improve the synthesis of bile in the liver, dissolve tiny gallstones, and treat chronic gastritis and other digestive system disorders. Although there is no research to prove its effectiveness on the treatment of cataracts it is believed that it can cure cataracts.

What Are The Benefits Of Using/Consuming Prodigiosa?
Although most of the benefits of using or consuming Prodigiosa is not back by any research but the Mexicans have been using this plant for all the under-listed purpose:
1. It is used for the treatment of diabetes (type II).
2. It is used for the treatment of diarrhea.

3. It is used for the treatment of stomach pain.
4. It is used for the treatment of gallbladder disease.
5. It is used to enhance the digestion of fat and boosting of the digestive system healthiness.

What Are The Side Effects Of Using/Consuming Prodigiosa?

Till at the time of writing this book, there are no side effects that have been recorded by people who have used or consume this plant/shrub.

What Are The Note-Full Precaution To Beware Of Before Using/Consuming Prodigiosa?

The note-full precautions to beware of before using or consuming Prodigiosa includes:

1. Pregnant and breast-feeding mothers should not use or consume Prodigiosa as there is no research to back it if it is safe or not.
2. It is a no go area for people that are suffering from diabetes I. and people with diabetes II should control their sugar level while consuming this herb.
3. Because this herb can control your sugar level, it is recommended that you don't consume this herb two weeks before and after surgery.

What Are The Medications That Interact With Prodigiosa?

Since Prodigiosa has the potency to lower blood sugar levels, consuming any diabetes medication alongside Prodigiosa will interact, thereby leading to an over-lowered blood sugar level. Diabetes medications include:

- Insulin
- Rosiglitazone (Avandia)
- Glimepiride-rosiglitazone (Avandaryl)
- Glyburide (Glynase/ Micronase/PresTab/DiaBeta)
- Glimepiride (Amaryl)
- Glipizide (Glucotrol)
- Tolbutamide (Orinase/Tol-Tab)
- Glipizide-metformin (Metaglip)
- Pioglitazone (Actos)
- Chlorpropamide (Diabinese)

- Glimepiride-pioglitazone (Duetact)
- Glyburide-metformin (Glucovance)
- Gliclazide and others.

What Is The Dosage And How To Prepare Prodigiosa Tea/Infusion?

For the dosage and how to prepare Prodigiosa tea/infusion, kindly take the following steps:

i.   You can get some fresh prodigiosa leave from a nursery garden, or you can make an order online.

ii.   Dry the fresh leaves until it is dried.

iii. Once the fresh leaves are dried or the one you ordered for is available, boil 8 or 16ounce of water and brew 1 or 2 tablespoons of Prodigiosa leaves in the warm water for 15minutes.

iv.   After brewing it, strain the Prodigiosa leaves.

v.   For the dosage, take a cup (8ounce) of prodigiosa tea/infusion two times per day.

What Is Burdock Root?

Burdock root is the root of a delicious plant called Burdock that all its body or parts are useful as either food or medicine. This plant is called different names by different people. However, some of it names include: Burr Seed, Gobo, Arctium, Arctium tomentosum, Cocklebur, Grande Bardane, Bardane Comestible, Beggar's Buttons, Fox's Clote, Cockle Buttons, Edible Burdock, Bardane Majeure, Glouteron, Bardana, Great Bur, Arctium minus, Bardane Géante, Clotbur, etc. this plant can be found in all over the world. I called this plant the wonder plant because everything about it is important as we consume its root as food, and we also use it for medicinal purpose, and both its leaf and seed are used for medicinal purposes as well.

For over five centuries, people all over the world have been using burdock root orally to treat and prevent various health disorders.

How Does Burdock Root Work?

Because of the chemical composition of Burdock root, such as; quercetin and luteolin, research has it that it can serve as a great an effective anti-oxidants that can treat and prevent cancer by preventing cancerous cells from growing and mutating and also combat aging. The compound like 'Phytosterols' helps in boosting of scalp and hair follicles to grow healthy hair even from baldhead. The vitamins-C helps in boosting the immune system and combat bacterial. It also helps to cleanse or detoxify the liver and lymphatic system, etc.

The potassium helps in reducing blood sugar level and helps to filter the blood by removing impurities through the bloodstream and eradicate toxins through the skin and urine.

What Are The Benefits Of Using/Consuming Burdock Root?

The benefits of using or consuming burdock root tea/infusion include:

i. It helps to cleanse/detox the liver and lymphatic system.
ii. It is used to treat and prevent diabetes by reducing blood sugar levels in the body.
iii. It helps to eliminate toxins from the body by inducing sweet and urine.
iv. It helps to purify the blood by removing heavy metals from the bloodstream.
v. It helps to treat various skin disorders and combat against aging.
vi. It helps to treat and prevent cancer by inhibiting the growth and mutation of cancerous cells.
vii. It helps to boost the immune system and enhance circulation.
viii. It helps to treat some ailment like; fever, fluid retention, cold, arthritis, sexually transmitted disease, stomach upset, anorexia and aid in boosting of sexual urge (libido)

What Are The Side Effects Of Using Or Consuming Burdock Root?

Till at the time of writing this book, there are no side effects that have been recorded by researchers or people that have used these herbs.

However, research has it that applying this root to your skin might cause rashes.

What Are The Medications That Interact With Burdock Root?

Because of the fact that Burdock root has the potency to slow down blood clotting, any medication that does the same potency will certainly interact with Burdock root. Such medications are:

1. Anticoagulant/Antiplatelet medication/drug
2. Aspirin

3. Heparin
4. Warfarin (Coumadin)
5. Clopidogrel (Plavix)
6. Dalteparin (Fragmin)
7. Enoxaparin (Lovenox)
8. Diclofenac (Cataflam, Voltaren)
9. Ibuprofen (Motrin, Advil)
10. Naproxen (Naprosyn, Anaprox) etc.

What Is The Dosage And How To Prepare Burdock Root Tea/Infusion?

For the dosage and how to prepare Burdock root tea/infusion, kindly take the following steps:

1. Uproot some burdock root from a nursery farm or garden.
2. ii. Scrub the uprooted root of burdock heartily under running water to remove all the dirt that accompanied it from the soil.
3. You should chop the Burdock root into smaller pieces (less than 1 inch). Please note that if you order it online, it will come dried and already chopped.
4. Pour 2-3 cup of water into your saucepan and add ¼ cup of the chopped burdock root and boil it.
5. Once the water is boiling, lower your gas and re-boil it for a period of 30-40 minutes and put off your gas.
6. Once it is cold, strain it and consume it.
7. For the dosage, 1glass cup daily

What Is Dandelion?

Dandelion is a flowering plant, also known as; Taraxacum officinale, Lentodon taraxacum, cankerworm, clock flower, common dandelion, yellow gowan, piss-in-bed, priest's crown, pissinlit, puffball, lion's tooth, blow-ball, etc. This plant is a native to Eurasia, and today. It is common in over 60 countries all over the world in the mild climates of the northern hemisphere. For centuries, these flowering plants have been used for the treatment of swelling (inflammation) of the pancreas, relieve pains that is caused by inflammation, treat and prevent cancer, tonsils (tonsillitis), skin disorder, bladder or urethra disorder, digestive and liver problems and enhance the general health of the liver and digestive system.

How Does Dandelion Works?

Because of the chemicals compositions and nutrient like; vitamin-A, B, C, E and K, mineral-like; calcium, iron, magnesium and potassium and another compound like; Chicoric, Chlorogenic acid, and Polyphenols, that Dandelion contains, researchers proved that it is a very effective cleansing/detoxification herbs that can detoxify or cleanse; gallbladder, kidney and purifies blood by eliminating of heavy metals in the blood stream and increase the rate of urine production which will lead to the cleansing of the urinary tract and inhibit crystals from forming in the urine, dissolves kidney stones and enhance kidney's health, treat and prevent diabetes by regulating blood sugar level, relief liver and urinary disorder by enhancing the healthiness of the liver.

What Are The Benefits Of Using/Consuming Dandelion?

The benefits of using or consuming Dandelion include:

1. It is an effective detoxifying herb that helps to detoxify or cleanse the liver and the kidney.
2. ii. It helps to treat and prevent diabetes by regulating blood sugar levels.
3. It helps to fight against and relieve pains that are causedd by inflammation.
4. It helps to deactivate and inhibit the negative effects of free radicals in the body, which is because of its anti-oxidant properties.
5. It helps to reduce the level of cholesterol.
6. It helps to lower blood pressure by getting rid of excess fluid in the body.
7. It helps to naturally shed excess weight gain by improving the metabolism of carbohydrates.
8. It helps to prevent and treat cancer by inhibiting the growth and cancer cell mutation.
9. It helps in boosting the digestive system.
10. It helps to boost the immune system.
11. It helps to keep the skin healthy and treat and prevent skin diseases.

What Are The Side Effects Of Using Or Consuming Dandelion?

Till at the time of writing this book, consuming of Dandelion orally is 100% safe, but consuming overdose of dandelion can result in some side effects like:

1. Diarrhea
2. ii. Experiencing stomach upset or irritation
3. Allergic reactions
4. Sometimes heartburn, but it's not common.

What Are The Notable Precaution Before Using/Consuming Dandelion?

The notable precautions before using/consuming dandelions are:

1. Pregnant and breast-feeding mothers should stay off dandelion as there is no research to know if it is harmful to them or not.
2. ii. If you are suffering from Eczema, stays off dandelion as more than 85% of people with eczema suffer an allergic reaction to dandelion.
3. Since dandelion slows down blood clotting, people that have any history of bleeding disorders should stay of Dandelion as it might increase the risk of bleeding and bruising.
4. If you are allergic to other related plants from the same family like; marigolds, ragweed, chrysanthemums, or daisies, you should stay of dandelion.
5. If you have a history of any kind of kidney disorder or failure, stay off dandelion.

What Are The Medications That Interact With Dandelion?

Because of the potency of dandelion, there are medications that interact with it. Such medications are:

All antibiotics. Examples of antibiotic are;

1. Quinolone
2. Grepafloxacin (Raxar)
3. Ciprofloxacin (Cipro)
4. Trovafloxacin (Trovan)
5. Norfloxacin (Chibroxin or Noroxin)
6. Parfloxacin (Zagam)
7. Enoxacin (Penetrex) etc.
   a. Lithium: just like lithium, dandelion also has water pill or "diuretic." Effects and so, consuming both medications will lead to a decrease in the rate at which the body gets rid of lithium.

    b. Medications that are changed by the liver: any medications that can be changed by the liver will interact with dandelion. Such medication are:

8. Amitriptyline (Elavil)
9. Atorvastatin (Lipitor)
10.   Diazepam (Valium)
11.   Digoxin
12.   Entacapone (Comtan)
13.   Haloperidol (Haldol)
14.   Irinotecan (Camptosar)
15.   Lamotrigine (Lamictal)
16.   Propranolol (Inderal)
17.   Theophylline
18.   Verapamil (Calan/Isoptin) etc.

What Are The Dosage And How To Prepare Dandelion Tea/Infusion?

For the dosage and how to prepare Dandelion tea/infusion, kindly take the following steps:

1. Get some fresh leaves of dandelion and washed it under running water to remove all the dirt.
2. After washing it, pour ½ - 1 cup of the washed dandelion in your saucepan.
3. You should boil 4-5 cups of water and pour the boiled water inside the saucepan where you pour the dandelion and cover it for 12-15 hours or throughout the night (overnight) for it to get infuse properly.
4. By the next day, strain out the dandelion leaves, and you will be left with the dandelion tea/infusion.
5. For the dosage, take ½ tablespoon of Dandelion per ¾ cup of water 3 times daily. And if you ordered your dandelion online, you can take 4-10 grams of dry leaf of dandelion 3 times daily.

What Is Elderberry?

Elderberry is a dark purple berry from the elder tree also known as Elderberries, European Black Elderberry, European Elder Fruit, European elderberry, Sambucus Baccae, black elder, Arbre de Judas, Black-Berried Alder, Black Elderberry, Sureau Noir, Sussier, etc. this plant is a flowering plant from the family of Adoxaceae and native to Europe. Both the leaves and fruit (berries) of elderberry have been used for centuries now for the treatment of pain and swelling arising from inflammation. It also helps to stimulate urine production and induce sweat to detoxify the body system.

How Does Elderberry Works?

Because of how rich elderberry is with various compounds and nutrients like vitamin-C, dietary fiber, phenolic acids which is a great and powerful anti-oxidants that helps to prevent and decrease the damage that is causedd by oxidative stress in the body, it also contains some compound like flavonols such as kaempferol, quercetin, isorhamnetin and anthocyanins which gives the fruit the black-purple color and makes it a strong anti-oxidant and anti-inflammation agent. Elderberry also contains some nutrients like; calories, carbs, a minute amounts of protein and fat, and anthocyanins, which makes the plant to be a strong and effective anti-oxidant with anti-inflammatory properties.

What Are The Benefits Of Using/Consuming Elderberry?

The benefits of using/consuming elderberry include:

i.   It helps to treat and prevent cancer by inhibiting cancer cells mutation and destroying the cancerous cells in the body.
ii. It helps to cleanse and detoxify the lungs and respiratory system by eliminating mucus from the upper respiratory system and the lungs.
iii. It helps to treat constipation.
iv. It helps to treat flu and cold in less than 24hours.
v.   It helps to combat harmful bacteria in the body by preventing the growth of bacterial through its anti-bacterial properties.
vi. It helps to boost and support the immune defense system by increasing white blood cell production.
vii. It helps to protect and keep the skin healthy.
viii. It helps to relieve chronic fatigue syndrome and depression etc.

What Are The Possible Side Effects Of Using/Consuming Elderberry?

Till at the time of writing this book, there are no record of any side effects from researchers and people who have use elderberry but because of the compound that are presents in elderberry, it will be wise to use it for not more than 12weeks and take a break for at least a week before using it again.

What Are The Notable Precaution For Using Or Consuming Elderberry?

The notable precautions before using elderberry include;

i. Make sure children below 12 years do not use/consume elderberry, and children above 12, and less than 18 should not use it for more than 10days.

ii. Since there is no reliable information to know if elderberry is safe or not for pregnant and breast-feeding mothers, I strongly advise that they should stay off elderberry.

iii. People that have a history or suffering from an auto-immune disease like; multiple sclerosis, lupus, rheumatoid arthritis, etc. should stay off elderberry as it has the potency to boost the immune system to become more active which could worsen their situation.

What Are The Medications That Interact With Elderberry?

Since elderberry has the potency to increase or boost the immune defense system, any medications that are designed to decrease the function of the immune system will certainly interact with Elderberry. Such medications include:

i. Azathioprine (Imuran)
ii. ii. Sirolimus (Rapamune)
iii. Basiliximab (Simulect)
iv. Mycophenolate (CellCept)
v. Corticosteroids (glucocorticoids)
vi. Prednisone (Deltasone, Orasone)
vii. Daclizumab (Zenapax)
viii. Muromonab-CD3 (Orthoclone OKT3, OKT3), etc.

What Is The Dosage And How To Prepare Elderberry Tea/Infusion?

For the dosage and how to prepare Elderberry tea/infusion, kindly take the steps below:

1. Boil 8~12oz of water in your saucepan.
2. Once the water is boiling, measure one tablespoon of dried elderberries and add it to the boiling water.
3. Reduce your gas and allow it to boil for at least 15 minutes.
4. After the 15 minutes timing, allow it to get cold and strain it using a strainer.
5. For the dosage, consume 3~4 cups daily.

What Is Guaco?

Guaco is a climbing plant with different names like Cipo caatinga, Huaco, Guace, vejuco, Vedolin, bejuco, Cepu, Bejuco de finca, Liane Francois, etc. This climbing plant belongs to the family of Asteraceae and cordifolia species and is very rich with numerous minerals and compounds. Its leaves are very medicinal and nutritional, that the people of Aztecs use it for cleansing the blood system and clearing of heavy metals from the bloodstream. The leaves is also used to eliminate mucus/phlegm by increasing urine production, heals wound quickly, reduce inflammation, promote healthy respiration and perspiration, boost digestive health, treat and prevent venereal diseases, eliminate harmful bacteria from the body, relieve pain that is causedd by inflammation, thin blood and a lot more.

How Does Guaco Works?

Because of the various chemicals and minerals compound that Guaco contains like; Coumarin, Tannins, Cinnamoylgrandifloric acid, Kaurenoic acid, gain, Lupeol acetate o-hydroxy-cinnamic acid, stigmasterol etc. research has it that, these compound helps to make Guaco a very effective and efficient detoxifier as it helps to cleanse/detoxify the blood by clearing heavy metals from the blood, remove mucus/phlegm, heals wounds (both internal (ulcer) and external wound) and increase the production of urine and induce sweat to cleanse the entire body system. However, the leaves, when consuming as tea/infusion, also helps to boost the health of the digestive system, promote healthy respiration and perspiration, treat and prevent venereal diseases and also help to reduce inflammation and pains, destroy harmful bacteria, thin blood and boost the immune system.

What Are The Benefits Of Using/Consuming Guaco?

There are a lot of benefits that one can benefit from using or consuming Guaco. Such benefits are:

1. It can be used to lessen the effect or symptoms of snake poison.
2. It is used to thin the blood through the activities of coumarin that it contains (anticoagulant and blood-thinning.)
3. It helps to combat inflammation though its ant-inflammatory properties.
4. It helps to treat stomach irritation through the effect of its cleansing activities.
5. It helps to treat respiratory disorders like; coughs rheumatism, bronchitis, etc.
6. It helps to enhance quick recovery from the wound.
7. It helps to cleanse or detoxify the blood and skin by clearing heavy metal from the blood.
8. It helps to boost and build the immune defense system.
9. It helps to treat some infections disease such as; candida yeast infection, herpes, etc.

What Are The Side Effects Of Using Or Consuming Guaco?

Till at the time of writing this book, there are no severe side effects that researchers or uses have recorded that one can suffer from the used or consumption of Guaco, but there are moderate side effects like;

1. Diarrhea
2. Spewing
3. And lastly, nausea

What Are The Precaution To Be Note-Full Of Before Using/Consuming Guaco?

Like I said earlier, Guaco is 100% safe for consumption by mouth, but if you are taking or using any Coumadin drugs, please consult with your doctor before using it.

And if you have any history of bleeding, do not use Guaco unless your doctor approves of it.

Do not use Guaco two weeks before and after surgery.

What Are The Medications That Interact With Guaco?

Like I said earlier, Guaco helps to thin blood so any medications that can thin blood or slow blood clotting do interacts with Guaco. Such medications are:

1. Anticoagulant/Antiplatelet medication/drug
2. Aspirin
3. Heparin
4. Warfarin (Coumadin)
5. Clopidogrel (Plavix)
6. Dalteparin (Fragmin)
7. Enoxaparin (Lovenox)
8. Diclofenac (Cataflam, Voltaren)
9. Ibuprofen (Motrin, Advil)
10. Naproxen (Naprosyn, Anaprox) and others.

What Is The Dosage And How To Prepared Guaco Tea/Infusion?

For the dosage and how to prepare Guaco tea/infusion, kindly take the following steps:

1. Get some handful of fresh Guaco and wash it under running water or 2 ounces of it dried leaves if you have the dried ones.
2. Pour about 6cups of water in your saucepan together with the Guaco leaves boil it until it is reduced to 2 cups.
3. You can add some brown sugar (optional) if you add the brown sugar; allow it to boil for another 20 minutes.
4. Strain the syrup with a strainer.
5. You should bottled it and store it in a refrigerator.
6. For Guaco dosage, take 1 soup-spoon 3-4 times daily.

What Is Eucalyptus Tree?

Eucalyptus tree is a fast-growing evergreen tree that is a native of Australia. The leaves and bark of this plant is used for various medicinal purposes like for the treatment of; joint and muscle pain, cold, cough, congestion, etc. However, the Chinese, Greek, and Indian Ayurvedic people have incorporated this amazing herb for the treatment of various types of conditions for thousands of years before now. This plant/tree has more than 400 different species. The most used is the Eucalyptus globulus or the Australian fever tree, which is also known as Blue Gum.

How Does Eucalyptus Work?

Eucalyptus leaves contains cineole that is also known as eucalyptol, in which the leaf's gland contain an essential oil (eucalyptus oil) and also; flavonoids and tannins, which are plant-based anti-oxidants that aids in reducing inflammation, control blood sugar, fight against the activities of bacteria and fungi and the oil can help in relieving pain and inflammation as well as blocking chemicals that usually cause asthma.

What Are The Benefits Of Using Or Consuming Eucalyptus Tea/Infusion?

The benefits of using or consuming eucalyptus tea/infusion include:

1. It helps in cleansing the skin through steaming/sauna.
2. ii. Eucalyptus helps in relieving of common cold symptoms like: cough lozenges and inhalants and also, sore throat and sinusitis
3. It helps in relieving symptoms of bronchitis. In fact, inhaling the vapor of eucalyptus tea helps serves as a decongestant by loosening phlegm and easing of congestion.
4. It aids in relieving of asthma: research showed that, eucalyptus has the potency to break up mucous in people that are suffering from asthma.
5. It aids in dental plaque and improve gingivitis: research carried out on eucalyptus shows that, eucalyptus leaf has the potency to reduce dental plaque and improve gingivitis.
6. It helps in improving bad breath: research showed that eucalyptus has the potency to improve bad breath.
7. It also helps to relives some health like; skin disease, bladder diseases, gallbladder and liver problems, bleeding gums, diabetes, burns, ulcer, stuffy nose, wounds, etc.

What Are The Side Effects Of Consuming Or Using Eucalyptus Tea/infusion?

Until at the time of writing this book, eucalyptus leaves are 100% safe for consumption (amount in food).

However, the use of eucalyptus oil is not as safe as the leaves as applying the oil directly to the skin without being diluted can lead to serious nervous system problems.

What Are The Note-Full Precaution Of Using Eucalyptus Tea/Infusion?

The precaution to be note-full of before using eucalyptus tea or infusion include:

1. It is 100% safe for pregnant and breastfeeding mothers to consume eucalyptus tea/infusion, but the oil is completely unsafe.
2. The tea is safe for children, but the oil might lead to seizures or even death.
3. Because of the potency of eucalyptus leaves to lower blood sugar levels, it is advisable to consult with your doctor before using the tea with any diabetes medication as it can over lower blood sugar levels.
4. If you are allergic to it oil, you might want to take some caution in consuming the tea as it might react to you.
5. Before or after surgery, avoid consuming the tea of the eucalyptus tree for two weeks as your blood sugar level might not be controlled.

What Are The Medications That Interact With Eucalyptus?

Since the leaf of eucalyptus has the potency to lower blood sugar, consuming of any diabetes medication can interact with eucalyptus tea/infusion. Check such medications under medications that interact with Prodigiosa.

What Is The Dose And How To Prepare Eucalyptus Tea/Infusion?

For the dosage and how to prepare eucalyptus tea/infusion, kindly take the following steps:

1. Boil water to (90~95)° or 194~205 Fahrenheit. Alternatively, you can boil the water and drop it down for a minute or two to reduce the temperature.
2. Pour a teaspoon of dried eucalyptus leaf into a teacup/mug.
3. Pour 6 ounce of water (from the first step) inside the teacup/mug and allow the leaves to be steep for 10~15minutes. (you can enjoy breathing the vapors of the steeping tea)
4. Get a filter to strain the loose leaves of the eucalyptus.
5. You are a god. You can now enjoy the cup of the eucalyptus tea/infusion at a go.
6. For the dosage, take 3~4 cups per day.

Dr. Sebi Approved Herbs For

Hypertension Revitalization

How Do I Break My Fast After The Cleansing Period?
During the first three days of liquid or water fasting, your digestive system will shut-down. Once your digestive system is shut down, all your energy will be focus on healing as there is no food to direct energy to digest. To break your water or liquid fast, you will need to introduce solid food to your system slowly. If not, you might suffer from digestion issues. So, the first thing to do is to start eating fruits like watermelons and berries because they have a high level of water. To make it easier, consume fruit after every 3 days of your fast. After introducing the high water level fruit, you will now have to introduce banana and apple before you can try solid food.

Please note that if you are observing fruit or raw veggies fast, you won't need this step.

What Are The Revitalizing/Electrical Plants To Revitalize My Body For Hypertension?

Aside from the disease that will absorb your energy, when observing the fast/cleansing period, your body will be weak without much energy and disease because the food we eat is what leads to the compromising of the mucous membrane. To regain back that alkaline state (healthy body system), you will need to revitalize your body system to it healthy state by rejuvenating all the lost energy.

The revitalizing/electrical plants that you need to revitalize your body system after cleansing for hypertension are;

1. Flor De Manita: this herb helps to regulate blood pressure, support and improve cardiovascular health and ensure cholesterol level is maintained in the body system.

2. Lily Of The Valley: this is an amazing herb that is very rich in iron, phosphate, and potassium. It serves as a diuretic for kidney stones and as an effective tonic for the treatment of the central nervous system.

3. Herbal Del Sapo is another revitalizing herb that is used to lower blood sugar level and triglycerides, reduces weight naturally, cleanses the arteries, dissolves kidney stones, and other kidneys disorder.

4. Shepherd's purse: this revitalizing herb is a hemostatic diuretic and an astringent that has the potency to treat uterine bleeding, bladder infections, lower blood pressure, bleeding disorder, kidney disease, mild heart failure, etc.

5. Flor De Tila: this amazing herb is used for the treatment of rapid heartbeat, insomnia, incontinence, muscle spasms, stop excessive bleeding, lower high blood pressure, etc.

6. Sarsaparilla root: these cleansing herbs are the best source of iron for healing that helps in purifying the blood and center on getting rid of various infections disease, treat and prevent congestive heart failure, lower high blood pressure, urinary disorder, hive, impotence, PMS, infertility, inflammation, nervous disorder, etc.

7. Valerian root: this is another revitalizing herb that has the potency to lower blood pressure, migraine headache, hypochondria, anxiety, asthma, etc.

8. Yarrow: this herb helps in purifying the body system by inducing sweat, relieve gastrointestinal ailment, lower blood pressure, stop bleeding including heavy menstrual bleeding, coronary, cerebral, thrombosis, improve circulation, etc.

9. Lupulo: this herb helps break up calcification, calm the nervous system, treat insomnia, lower blood pressure and cholesterol, hot flashes, relieve pain, etc.

What Is Flor De Manita?

Flor De Manita is the flower that grows on sthe evergreen flowering tree genus belonging to the Malvaceae family. It is a native of Central and South American and can grow up to 50 feet tall.

The tree is called different names by different people. It names include macpalxochitl, hand flower tree, devil's hand tree, canaco, mecapalxochitl, mapilxochitl, berdonces, canahue, mexican handplant, cacpalxochitl, papasuchil, camxochitl etc. the bark, leaves, and flower of this tree are used for over a century for medicinal purpose for the treatment of various health disorder.

How Does Flor De Manita Works?

Because of the chemicals compound that Flor De Manita contains like: luteolin, alkaloids, and glycosides quercetin, which makes it to be an effective diuretics, pain reliever, anti-cholinergic and stimulant for heart problems. Because of its properties, research has it that this herb is a very effective remedy for various disorders like depression, nervousness, insomnia, epilepsy, inflammation, headache, ulcers, and piles. However, this herb is also used to treat afflictions affecting the pubic area and hemorrhoids. Finally, it helps to treat gastrointestinal diseases like; diarrhea and dysentery

What Are The Benefits Of Using/Consuming Of Flor De Manita?
The benefits of using/consuming of Flor De Manita include:
i.   It is used to regulate blood pressure.
ii.   ii. It is used as a stimulant for various heart disorders.
iii.   It is used to lower abdominal pain.
iv.   It is used to reduce edema and serum cholesterol levels.
v.   It is used to relieve and sooth pains arising from inflammation.
vi.   It is used to regulate and normalized bowel function
vii.   It helps to supports and improves cardiovascular health.
viii. It is used to treat epilepsies.
ix.   It is also used for the treatment of gastrointestinal infections like dysentery and diarrhea.

What Are The Side Effects Of Using/Consuming Of Flor De Manita?
Till at the time of writing this book, there are no side effects that have been reported by researchers and users of this herb. Therefore, this herb is 100% safe for consumption.

What Are The note-full Precautions Before Using Flor De Manita?
The note-full precautions before using Flor De Manita include:
i.   Because there is no sufficient information with respect to the negative effect of this herb on pregnant and breastfeeding mothers, I will advise that they stay safe and avoid using it.
ii.   ii. If you are on anti-hypertensive or anti-epileptic medications, talk to your doctor before using this herb.

What Are The Medications That Interacts With Floe De Manita?

Medication that interacts with Flor De Manita includes:

1. Any medications made for hypertension: since Flor De Manita has the potency to lower high blood pressure and all hypertension medications have the same potency, if these two medications are consumed together, there are tendencies that you might suffer low blood pressure. Such medications include:

   - ACE inhibitors
   - Alpha-blockers
   - Alpha-2 Receptor Agonists
   - Angiotensin II receptor blockers
   - Beta-blockers
   - Central agonists
   - Combined alpha and beta-blockers
   - Calcium channel blockers
   - Diuretics
   - Peripheral adrenergic inhibitors
   - Vasodilators

2. Any epileptic medications: since Flor De Manita has the potency to treat the nervous disorder and epileptic medications do the same, consuming both medications will interact. Such medications include:

   - Topiramate (Topamax)
   - Zonisamide (Zonegran)
   - Carbamazepine (Tegretol/Carbatrol etc)
   - Valproic acid (Depakene)
   - Phenobarbital
   - Lamotrigine (Lamictal)
   - Gabapentin (Neurontin/Gralise) etc

What Is The Dosage And How To Prepare Flor De Manita?

For the dosage and how to prepare Flor De Manita Tea/Infusion, kindly take the steps below:

1. Get some flowers of the Flor De Manita or the leaves and dry it. You can order it online, and it will come dried and chopped.

2. Boil a cup (8~10ounce) of water.
3. Once the water is boiling, add 1 tablespoon of Flor De Manita
4. Allow it to boil for 10~15 minutes.
5. Put off the fire and allow it to get cool.
6. Strain it, and you are done. For the dosage, consume a cup (8~10ounce) 3times daily.

What Is Lily Of The Valley?

Lily of the valley is an amazing flowering plant that both the root, underground stem (rhizome), and dried flower tips are used for medicinal purposes. This flowering plant is also known as: muguet. This plant has been used traditionally for centuries for the treatment and preventions of a lot of health problems.

How Does Lily Of The Valley Work?

Because of the chemicals and compound that lily~of~the~valley contains, research shows that this flowering plant has the potency to stimulate heart muscle contractions, induce labor which can lead to miscarriage, stabilize heartbeat and excitability, improve the health of the heart and prevent heart failure, treat and prevent urinary tract infections (UTIs), kidney disorder, epilepsy, edema, eye infection, paralysis, strokes etc.

What Are The Benefits Of Using/Consuming Lily Of The Valley?

The benefits of using or consuming lily of the valley include:
1. It is used to treat and prevent heart disorders like irregular heartbeat, heart failure, etc.
2. It is used to treat and prevent urinary tract infections (UTIs).
3. It is used to boost the health of the kidney and dissolve kidney stones.
4. It is used to stimulate contractions to induce labor.
5. It is used to treat epilepsy and fluid retention.
6. It is used to treat and prevent strokes and paralysis.
7. It is used for the treatment of eye infection (conjunctivitis).
8. It is used to treat and prevent leprosy etc.

What Are The Side Effects Of Consuming/Using Of Lily Of The Valley?

The possible side effects from using/consuming lily of the valley include:
1. Nausea
2. Spewing

3. Experience abnormal heartbeat.
4. Frequent headache
5. Reduces consciousness and rate of responsiveness
6. Reduces visual color disturbances etc.

What Are The Precautions To Beware Of Before Using/Consuming Of Lily Of The Valley?

The precautions to beware of before using/consuming lily of the valley include:

1. It is 100% unsafe for pregnant and nursing mothers to used lily of the valley without any medical supervision.
2. If you are suffering from heart disorder or you have a history of any heart disorder, don't use lily of the valley without close supervision from a medical practitioner.
3. If you are suffering from potassium deficiency, please do not use this herb as it will worsen the situation.

What Are The Medications That Interacts With Lily Of The Valley

Medications that interact with the lily of the valley include:

1. Since Lily-of-the-valley has the potency to stimulate the heart, any calcium supplement does the same, which might affect the heart and make it to be too stimulated.
2. Just like cascara sagrada, lily of the valley is very effective in decreasing potassium levels in the body; and digoxin does the same thing, combining the two medications together will lead to potassium deficiency from the body system
3. Any drugs that are made for inflammation interact with lily of the valley. You can check for such medications under medications that interact with Cascara Sagrada.
4. Lily of the valley interacts with Quinine as both medications have the same potency to affect the heart.
5. Some anti-biotic and medications that have a water pill or diuretic effect might interact with lily of the valley, so consult with your doctor before combining any of these medications.

What Is The Dosage And How To Prepare Lily Of The Valley Tea/Infusion?

For the dosage and how to prepare lily of the valley tea/infusion, kindly take the following steps:

1. Harvest some fresh lily of the valley leaves by uprooting it.
2. Wash it under running water and dry it afterward.

3. Once it is dried, chopped it into smaller pieces or pounds it. Alternatively, you can order for it online, and it will come dried and chopped.
4. Once it is dry, it is ready to use.
5. Measure 1teaspoons of the chopped dried lily of the valley and pour it in a teacup/mug.
6. Boil 8 ounces of water and pour it into the teacup or mug with the dried lily of the valley and allow it to steep for 15minutes.
7. Strain it using a strainer or filter.
8. For the dosage, take 1cup (8ounce) 2-3 times daily.

CONCLUSION OF "THE DR. SEBI TREATMENTS AND CURES"

T hank you for making it through to the end of Dr. Sebi's treatments and cure. Let's hope it was informative and able to provide you with all of the tools you need to achieve your goals whatever they may be.

It was here that Dr. Sebi's diet was born. He learned that if he ensured that the body remained in an alkaline state, diseases would not thrive. Diseases need acid to live and grow. Although his diet requires that he cut out a lot of food, many people have had success with his teachings. This book is here to provide you with treatment to help you get started on the Dr. Sebi diet. All nutrients follow your nutritional guide to let you know that you are not eating more than approved foods. All you have to do is decide which supplements to take.

The diet does not have to be complicated. Dr. Sebi makes your diet simple, effective, and satisfying. If you are serious about your health, choosing this book will be one of the best decisions you can make. Maybe you already know Dr. You and Sebi are looking for an easy way to get started. Even if you are not sure who it is, this book will guide you in the right direction.

Many people claim that his diet improved their health by using his compounds, and the herbal approach to heal the body worked better than any medical approach ever did. You can find many of his thoughts about herbal therapy and nutritional compounds on YouTube that help promote and teach healthy living long after his death.

Diets that are rich in fruits and vegetables are associated with oxidative stress and reduced inflammation, along with protecting you against most diseases.

Meatless diets have been linked to lower risks of heart disease and obesity. It also encourages foods that are high in fiber and low in calories. Regularly consuming fruits and vegetables can help protect your body against diseases and reduce inflammation.

If you can switch from your normal diet that is full of fast foods, saturated fats, refined sugars, and grains to Dr. Sebi's diet could actually help you lose some weight—increasing your intake of whole grains, vegetables, and fruits while getting rid of pork and beef can decrease your risk of elevated cholesterol, high blood pressure, Type 2 diabetes, heart disease, and cancer. Most people eat way too much sodium, and this diet can reduce drastically lower this amount. This, in turn, can help you lower your blood pressure, and this reduces your risk of heart disease and stroke.

In one study, people who ate seven servings of fruits and vegetables each day had between a 25 and 31 percent lower chances of heart disease and cancer.

Most Americans don't eat enough produce. During 2017 it was reported that between 9.3 and 12.2 percent met all their recommended daily intake of fruits and vegetables.

Dr. Sebi's diet encourages eating healthy fats like plant oils, seeds, and nuts along with whole grain that is rich in fiber. These foods have a lower risk of developing heart disease.

Any diet that limits processed foods can help you have a better quality of diet.

INTRODUCTION OF "THE DR. SEBI DIET"

A lfredo Darrington Bowman, also known as Doctor Sebi, was a Honduran herbalist, pathologist, naturalist, and biochemist. He studied and observed different herbs in Africa, South and Central America, the Caribbean, and North America. After many years of empirical research and experience, he developed a unique methodology for curing the human body with herbs and a specialized diet.

This diet is called the Doctor Sebi Diet. The Doctor Sebi Diet has helped many people suffering from chronic diseases feel better without taking pills. Doctor Sebi developed the diet for those who wish to prevent or cure disease naturally and improve their health without relying on standard Western medicine.

He claimed that plant-based meals had the potential to help people prevent diseases, and they could serve as treatment plans for chronic medical conditions such as diabetes. The diet is based on vegetables and other plants that are able to create an alkaline environment in the body.

Doctor Sebi believed that high acidity levels promote pathogen development and create an environment that fosters the creation of disease-causing mucus. For instance, pneumonia is caused by mucus accumulation in the lungs, while diabetes is a result of excess mucus in the pancreas.

This diet reduces drastically the contamination of the body and encourages an overall wellbeing. If you decide to follow this life-changing diet, you will not also develop better and safer eating strategies, but curb the occurence of other typical chronic diseases.

If you need to lose weight, this diet motivates you to do it easily and reliably. But it is not about losing weight, but rather itt's about improving the strength and endurance that everyone needs.

There is more to the alkaline diet than meets the eye. A few short sentences are not enough to detail everything you need to know about it. This is why, in this book, we are going to explore in details the claims made by Dr. Sebi and the scientifical basis of his diet.

This book also presents the original Dr. Sebi recipes to plan all your meals, including the different ingredients and the steps involved in the preparation of the meal. You will always have a wide choice of yummy recipes to pick from for every meal, so that you will spend less time brainstorming on what to eat, and make it easier to adhere to the alkaline healthy living lifestyle.

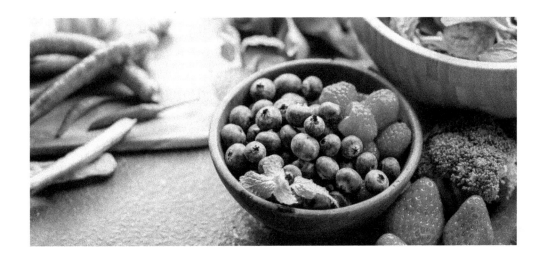

CHAPTER 37

Benefits of Dr. Sebi's Medicine

Reduce the risk of hypertension and stroke

A great benefit of eating an alkaline diet is the reduction of the risk of stroke and hypertension an individual is prone to have. A typical alkaline diet has an anti-aging effect. A robust result of the anti-aging effects is that it drastically reduces inflammation and fosters the growth of hormone production. This has been verified to help in the improvement of cardiovascular health and giving the body defense against typical health challenges like hypertension, high cholesterol, stroke, kidney stones, and possible memory loss.

Reduce chronic pain and inflammation

There is a correlation between alkaline diets and a drastic reduction in levels of chronic pain. Chronic acidosis is dangerous to the human health system. It is the primary cause of headaches, chronic back pain, joint pain, inflammation, menstrual symptoms, and muscle spasms.

Several studies show the health benefits of an alkaline diet for patients suffering from chronic pains. A study conducted showed that there was a significant level of decrease in the pain experienced by patients suffering from chronic back pain when they were given supplements containing alkaline daily for four weeks.

Give protection to bone density and muscle mass

Taking minerals into your body system plays a significant role in maintaining and developing the bones in your body. Research has proven beyond the shadow of a doubt that the more alkaline-rich fruits and vegetables you take regularly, the better you get protected from experiencing reduced bone muscle and strength known as Sarcopenia.

What an alkaline diet does when you take it is to help in balancing the ratios of the various minerals in the body necessary for the bone-building and the maintenance of a lean muscle mass. The minerals that an alkaline diet balances are Phosphate, Magnesium, and Calcium. Another benefit of an alkaline diet in this regard is the improvement in the production of vitamin D absorption and growth hormones, which helps in further protecting the bones and fighting against many chronic diseases.

Weight loss

This diet was not made with weight loss in mind, but because it is extremely restrictive, you will see weight loss. Also, one of the main reasons that this diet is effective in reducing weight is that it makes people stop consuming Western foods, which are highly caloric, oily, and sugary. Weight loss occurs when you eat less or equal amounts of calories that you can burn. If you follow this diet, which is low in sugar, fat, and processed foods, you can get your perfect body.

Improves kidney function

Acidic diets mostly affect the health of the kidneys and damages the layers inside the organ system. To promote kidney health, the pH of the urine mustn't be acidic. By consuming a lot of alkaline food and removing acidic foods from our daily routine, we can reach this pH in which our kidneys remain safe and healthy. Alkaline diets do not affect the pH of the blood, but it can significantly affect the urine. Drinking a lot of water alongside this diet can improve kidneys even more. If you're suffering from any chronic kidney disease, then you should know that this diet is not targeted for you. You can follow the diet after consulting your doctor first.

Reduces the risk of cancer

There are almost no significant studies that show that an alkaline diet leads to decreased cases of cancer. However, there have been studies that show that if a person were to eat less meat and increase their consumption of fresh fruits and vegetables, then that person is at a lower risk of cancer. Also, another study showed that having more vitamins, like vitamin C, in your diet can prevent cancer. Generally, eating more fruits and vegetables and consuming less high fatty and sugary foods leads to a reduction in developing cancer.

Reduces the risk of heart disease

Heart disease is the major cause of death in the world. It is mainly caused by eating lots of fat and oily foods, which results in the development of plaque and blockage of arteries. In this diet, the consumption of fats goes down significantly, decreasing the chances of developing heart disease. It has also been shown that growth hormones are related to decreased rates of heart disease. An alkaline diet increases the levels of growth hormones, so, in turn, it decreases heart disease as well.

Reduces the risk of muscle degradation

When we grow old or stop using our muscles, we tend to increase muscle loss. However, there was a study conducted in 2013 showing that people who follow the alkaline diet could decrease muscle degradation. The diet is low in red meat, so there is a risk of decreasing muscle mass and strength.

Increases intestinal health

With the addition of whole grains, there is a list of nuts and seeds that you can eat on this diet. It contributes to an increase in fiber intake, which increases the health of small and large intestines. It helps manage regular bowel movements, which reduces the risk of developing many diseases.

Decreases the harmful effects of processed foods

Processed foods have been linked to increased sugar intake and fat content. They also contain lots of calories but have very low nutritional value. Many additives and preservatives that have no purpose in our body are eliminated from our diets if we strictly avoid processed foods.

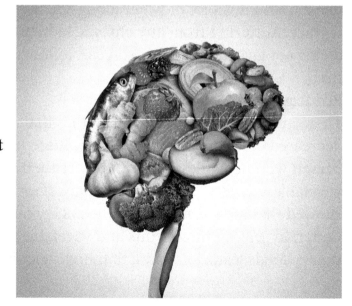

It helps the brain

The growth hormone is not only related to a better heart condition but also helps manage the health of the mind. It is related to an increase in memory and cognition. Eating a healthy diet rich in fruits and vegetables leads to better brain functioning.

It may improve back pain

Alkaline minerals are related to the reduction of back pain, but whether alkaline foods provide the same results has yet to be determined. There is a decent chance that the diet has similar effects.

Decreases the level of inflammation

Diets rich in fresh fruits and vegetables show a great decrease in oxidative stress and inflammation. This leads to less discomfort and fewer diseases developing in our bodies. Prevent deficiency in magnesium and increases vitamin absorption. Magnesium plays an essential role in the human body as an increase in its quantity is necessary for the proper functioning of all the enzymes and processes in the human body. Deficiency in magnesium content will result in headaches, anxiety, heart complications, muscle pains, and sleep troubles. Magnesium is also needed by the body in the activation of vitamin D and preventing Vitamin D deficiency, necessary for the functioning of the endocrine and overall body immunity.

Improving cancer protection and immune function

Minerals are needed by the body in disposing of waste or in oxygenating the body. But when there is a shortage of the required minerals in the cells, the body suffers. Vitamin absorption is zeroed off whenever there is a mineral loss in the body. Also, toxins and pathogens will pile up in the body, thereby weakening the immune system. But with alkaline diets, that cannot happen as research has proved that the death of cancerous cells happens more in an alkaline body. Alkaline diets will help in decreasing inflammation and the possible risks associated with dangerous diseases such as cancer.

Help you in maintaining a healthy balanced weight

When you eat more of alkaline diets, you are not just limiting the acidic content in your body but also protecting your body from the risks associated with obesity. This is possible as alkaline diets decrease the levels of Leptin and inflammation, which has a direct effect on your hunger and fat-burning capacities.

CHAPTER 38

How to Fast Properly with Dr. Sebi Diet

What Is Fasting?

The best way to safely fast is the question on the lips of many. Before we delve into that, there is a need to paint a clearer picture of what fasting is. Abstinence from food totally or partially for some reason is what is regarded as fasting. According to Dr. Alvenia Fulton, "The best juices are fresh juices made from your blender out of fresh fruits and vegetables, not from canned or frozen foods."

Before you fast;

#1. Fasting comes in two phases in order to cleanse your body effectively. Firstly, you have to cleanse your body with natural herbs for at least five days before embarking on the actual fasting.

#2. When you are ready for the fast, your body will give an indication of that,

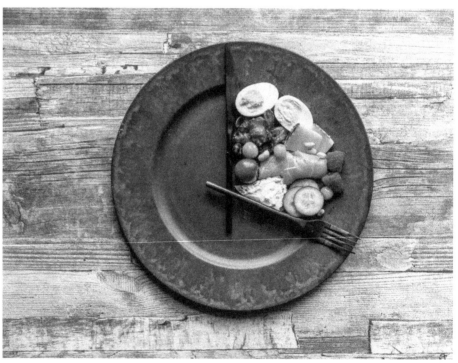

and the indication you are going to get is during the cleansing with herbs phase. When you start feeling hungry while cleansing is when you are truly ready to begin your fast. You should never fast when your body is not ready, if you feel hungry during a fast, you should eat.

Why should you fast

If you want to know how to correct your body's discomforts, fasting will fix your body and keep you younger. The best method of fasting is to clean the body until there is no more hunger. When there is no hunger, you can fast as long as you like. Fast until your appetite returns because it will disappear. The tongue will become white and soft; fast until the tongue turns red again, and fast until your breath and your body become sweet. The body will produce its own smell due to the removal of all the toxic waste in the body.

What fasting will do

You will look younger, feel younger, skin rejuvenated, and your hair and nails will be revitalized. Fasting will do all these things in your body. If you fast, your body will remain flexible, full of energy, and shine with vitality. This is what we all want, and nothing will do that better than cleansing and fasting. Nothing will do a better job at healing, developing, and relieving our body of waste and toxins if not for fasting (juice, vegetable, or water fasting).

What about Water fasting

Fasting with water is better because it will clean the body of toxic waste, heal the body of old dead cells that have been there for a long time. The best way to do this is to cleanse the body and then start the water fast. When you fast, you will find that your skin becomes resonant, young, and beautiful. Your hair, your eyes, and every gland in your body will respond to fasting.

This is what they all need, the intense cleansing that occurs from fasting. If you fast, your friends or people you know can say that you are killing yourself. But I did not listen to them; even during biblical days, people fasted for 21, 30, or 40 days, and no one died of fasting. The prophets, Jesus and the women of the Bible, fasted, and no one died for it. Queen Esther fasted and saved the children of Israel from extinction. Fasting is a way of life.

How to Prepare for Fasting

Your fasting should start with cleansing. Use different natural herbs for 3 to 5 days before starting your fast, be it a juice, a vegetable, or water fast. Take herbs first to remove some of the toxin and body waste.

Most people have toxins that have been in their bodies since they were babies, so herbs are very important before any type of fasting. For example, the first time I tried fasting, on the 21st day, I could not get up quickly enough to go to the bathroom because I had a lot of toxins coming out of me

How long should you fast?

After cleaning the body with herbs, fast for 21 or 30 days until you no longer have a "coated" tongue, you no longer feel tired, weak, or nervous and you feel young again. The people around you are going to ask you what you are doing; you will look more youthful. Then, break the fast and begin again; if you cleanse the body quickly and adequately, you do not need to take drugs to do what you want. Male or female, your sex drive will continue to work well, and your hormones will work if they are cleansed and quickly.

Fast to Cleanse Toxins

You will come to the realization that what keeps us alive as humans are not food. What keeps us alive is getting rid of toxins and waste in our body. When we consume what nature has provided us with, and we fast to cleanse our body on top of that, our body and mind will change.

Our ancestors do not have prostate glands problems like the young men of nowadays. Our grandmothers as well, did not lose their youthful factor as it is in today's world. As a matter of fact, my great grandmother had twin babies at the age of 49, but this is unheard of in the 21st century despite all the medical discoveries. When we eat according to what nature has in store for us, we will stay healthy, live longer, and every pain in the body will vanish. Good health will ultimately triumph when we cleanse our body and stick to the right diet.

How Do You Break a Fast?

You are to break a fast exactly the way you started. By this, I mean, get a juice, warm it up and take that for 5 consecutive days. You will have more energy than you need. You won't feel hungry. If you jump right into taking steaks after an extensive fasting period, you will get sick.

That food will make you fall ill. You have to totally stop all those kinds of food as they cause body pains and ache. You did not come to this world to live a short life. There are so many ways to fast. The aim of this guide and information therein is to know the correct way for you to fast. In the end, this is all about choosing a fasting method that works well for you.

Foods During Fasting

Dr. Sebi has recommended foods that are easy to digest and ones that will push the body's performance to its peak.

Basically, fasting is abstinence from food, and this act greatly improves the elimination of waste materials from the body. Pollution, environmental toxins, synthetic medication, electrical radiation are all forms of things we take that can diminish our overall health. Fasting is a mechanism that speedily removes toxins like mucus, fecal waste, parasites, and phlegm from the body.

What Type Of Fasting Foods To Eat

The world-renowned doctor, Dr. Sebi, recommends that if you have to eat during a fast for medical reasons, you must know the right combinations of food to eat that will further aid the elimination of wastes and toxins. It is more advantageous to eat natural alkaline fruits, vegetables, and freshly made juices from these fruits.

#1 To provide the elements that your body needs during a fast, there is a need to eat foods that are rich in minerals and can be easily broken down and digested by the body. This diet will ensure that your body has excess energy to expel waste materials before beginning its healing process.

Dr. Sebi Fasting Foods Checklist

Here are the benefits of Dr. Sebi's fasting food; these are the benefits to your body when you eat the recommended fasting foods. Natural foods all contain 92 minerals found in the soil of the earth, 27 of which are found and play an important role in the human body to restore good health and bring our body back to its original state of health. These foods contain the following benefits that are essential for the optimal and proper functioning of the body.

The fasting foods provide:
- ✓ Alkalinity
- ✓ Iron, calcium, magnesium, copper, zinc, and many other minerals
- ✓ Expel mucus
- ✓ Easy to digest, assimilate, and used by the body
- ✓ They flush out the body and detox harmful wastes
- ✓ Neutralize the body's PH balance
- ✓ Restore the body overall good health
- ✓ Get rid of toxins

The Fasting Foods to Eat
Fruits:
- Seeded melons
- Mangoes
- All types of berries
- Papaya and many more

Vegetables to Eat During Fasting
If you have to eat during your fast for medical reasons or any other situation you are in.
These vegetables are ideal for consumption because of their ability to help the body expel mucus or toxins due to their high mineral content:
- Dandelion leaves
- Green leafy vegetables
- Kale

CHAPTER 39

Downsides of the Dr. Sebi Diet

While Dr. Sebi diet is very helpful in improving one's health and can improve the quality of life of people, there can be a few downsides or cons to following the Dr. Sebi diet to the letter.

Restricted food intake

The Dr. Sebi diet is a modified vegan diet with supplement requirements, in essence. However, while vegan diets already tend to be very restrictive, the Dr. Sebi diet goes even further and has a lot more restrictions.

Not only are adherents required to avoid animal products altogether and rely wholly on plant-based foods like other vegans, but there are also further more specific restrictions. Standard vegan diets, for example, allow any fruit and simply set limits on consumption amounts.

The Dr. Sebi diet, however, goes as far as to bar one from eating certain types of fruit, such as Roma tomatoes or beefsteak tomatoes being restricted, while cherry and plum tomatoes are permitted.

This may lead to certain difficulties when adhering to the diet, as it has been shown that strict diets are more difficult to follow. As such, if one finds it difficult or impossible to follow the diet, then they will not be able to benefit from the diet in the first place, defeating the purpose of following the diet.

Reliance on Supplementation

While supplements are not an inherently bad thing, the Dr. Sebi diet needs one to take specific types of supplements, which can be expensive or hard to source, depending on where one is in the world.

Dr. Sebi diet supplements are necessary, but not exclusive, meaning that one should also be taking other supplements in order to make up for any vitamin deficiencies that might have popped up along the way.

This means that one may be confused as to what additional supplements may be necessary, and thus one who intends to start the Dr. Sebi diet should consult with a nutritionist in order to design their diet plan in adherence to the Dr. Sebi rules and to find out what additional supplements, if any, may be necessary. In addition, the fact that these supplements necessarily show the inherent flaw in a vegan-based diet, where relying only on plant-based products leads to nutrient deficiencies that need to be made up for using supplementation.

For example, protein tends to be hard to come by in vegan diets and even more so in Dr. Sebi's more restrictive version, and protein is an essential macronutrient for us to stay healthy. While nuts are a source of protein, it tends to be difficult and impractical to gain all the protein we need just through nut consumption, and thus the need for supplementation. Other things that need to be supplemented are for nutrients such as omega 3, iron, calcium, and vitamin B12, which are all necessary to keep the body healthy and balanced but will be difficult to come by when following the Dr. Sebi diet, and thus needing supplementation.

Risk Of Vitamin Deficiencies
One very important thing that we must remember that is while vegetables are extremely nutrient-dense, and are in fact the best sources for some of the essential nutrients.
Meaning that the body will not worry about getting these nutrients, there are some nutrients that cannot be provided by an all – plant matter diet, such as Vitamin B – 12, vitamin D, calcium, and certain fatty acids such as the long-chain Omega – 3 fatty acid commonly found in fish, as these nutrients cannot be created by the body using the building blocks it obtains from food, but rather must be obtained directly from an outside source, and one of the better sources and the most easily – absorbable sources, (bioavailable source) would be animal products. As such, vegans are recommended to supplement their diet using appropriate supplementation, in order to make sure that they get all the necessary nutrients to maintain their health and to make sure that they keep a balanced diet.
While supplements in the Dr. Sebi diet are crucial and are included in the diet design, the diet itself does not specify food portions and meal design, which means that the supplements may not be enough to make up for nutrient deficiencies that may occur.

As the Dr. Sebi diet does not necessarily prescribe what exactly to eat and just prescribes what may be eaten, some people may eat more of one thing and less of another, which may lead to nutrient imbalances, even with the inclusion of the necessary supplements.

One example of this, for example, would be B – 12 nutrient deficiency. Those who are predominantly vegetarian or vegan, and do not eat animal products are already at risk of developing a vitamin B – 12 deficiency, and thus are recommended to take supplements to cover it. The Dr. Sebi diet supplements may not give enough B – 12 vitamins that one needs, and this is not entirely clear, as the Dr. Sebi diet supplements are necessary, but not exclusive, meaning that one should also be taking other supplements in order to make up for any vitamin deficiencies that might have popped up along the way.

Without consulting a qualified nutritionist, one may run into the risk of developing deficiencies, and thus extra care should be taken when planning and designing a diet plan around Dr. Sebi's diet principles. Another nutrient that those who take the Dr. Sebi diet should watch out for is protein, as with any other vegan diet, protein tends to be in short supply, and should be made up for through supplementation.

FOODS TO EAT
As we discussed earlier, the Dr. Sebi diet is very strict as to what foods are allowed and what foods are not allowed or what should be avoided. This list can be very specific, and as such, will need to be discussed here.
Some specific foods included on a diet would be as follows:

Fruits
Not all fruits are permitted under the Dr. Sebi diet, and fruits that are allowed would be apples, currants, dates, elderberries, berries, peaches, pears, seeded key limes, figs, cantaloupe, mangoes, seeded melons, prickly pears, and tamarinds. Notably, non – seeded variants of fruits are not included in this list, as this would entail the usage of modified foods, which Dr. Sebi was not able to analyze, and such, given the unknown effects, they are to be avoided.

Vegetables

Similarly, not all vegetables are allowed to be consumed under the Dr. Sebi diet, and the list of permitted vegetables are as follows: avocado, cactus flowers, chickpeas, dandelion greens, lettuce (NOT iceberg lettuce), kale, bell peppers, cucumber, mushrooms (NOT shiitake), okra, sea vegetables, olives, squash, tomatoes (cherry and plum tomatoes ONLY), zucchini. Take note of the exceptions within the list, such as not eating iceberg lettuce, and the only tomato variants allowed being cherry and plum.

Grains

Fonio, Khorasan wheat, rye, wild rice, quinoa, spelt, amaranth are the allowed grains. Note that whole grains are encouraged here, and Kamut, or Khorasan wheat is the specific variant of wheat that is encouraged. Note as well that the grains here may take the form of pasta, bread, flour, or cereal, but leavened food is banned, preventing foods made with baking powder or yeast.

Nuts, Seeds, and Oils

Avocado oil, coconut oil (non - processed), grapeseed oil, Brazil nuts, hemp seeds, raw sesame seeds, raw tahini butter, walnuts, hempseed oil, olive oil (virgin /non-processed), sesame oil are the allowed nuts, seeds, and oils under the Dr. Sebi diet. Note that non – processed oils are allowed, as the processed oil version is banned.

Herbs and Spices

While the Dr. Sebi diet encourages, and in fact requires the consumption of water, at least one gallon a day, herbal teas are allowed. Herbal teas such as elderberry, fennel, tila, ginger, burdock, raspberry, tila, fennel, and chamomile are all allowed. Herbs and spices such as oregano, basil, bay leaf, dill, basil, achiote, habanero, cayenne, onions, tarragon, cloves, sage, sea salt, thyme, seaweed, agave syrup, and date sugar are all allowed as well. This allows one to create tasty and satisfying foods, even if one has a sweet tooth, as agave syrup and date sugar are allowed, though white sugar and cane sugars are not allowed.

CHAPTER 40

Transition to Alkaline Diet

The Alkaline Diet: Powerful Weight-Loss Plan

What if you heard of a reduction of weight plan to help you reduce weight and look younger? Will you try? Should you try it? Alkaline diets and behaviors have been around for more than 60 years, and many people don't know about their normal, healthy, and tested weight-loss properties!

The alkaline diet is not a fad or a gimmick. It is a safe and quick way to experience higher fitness rates. This section will inform you what this diet program is, what makes it special, and how it will result in life-changing outcomes for you, your tail, and your wellbeing.

Will you love today a lean and beautiful body? You are in the minority, if so. Unfortunately, more than 65% of Americans are overweight or obese. If you are overweight, it is possible that you suffer poor health conditions such as weakness, stiffness, swollen muscles, and a variety of other illnesses.

Worse still, you still have the impression that you still love the body you like and deserve. Maybe you were told you are growing older, but that's just not the truth. Don't give in to that myth. Don't fall into that myth. Many communities have strong, lean elderly people who go to great health in their 1990s!
The reality is that the body is a computer of a genius architecture, and if you experience some adverse health effects, that is proof that the blood composition is too acidic. The signs are a call for assistance. That is for one day; the body will not break down. Rather, your wellbeing is gradually eroding over time, finally slipping into 'disappointment.'

What's wrong with the way you're eating now?

The standard American Diet (S.A.D) relies on processed foods, fats, caffeine, meats, and animal goods. All of these products are extremely acidic. Although we consume not enough of the alkaline foods such as new fruits, vegetables, nuts, and legumes, given the appeals of diet experts.

In brief, our S.A.D. lifestyle upsets our species' normal acid-alkaline equilibrium. This illness induces malnutrition, higher rates of aches and pains, colds and flu, and disease inevitably develops.

We missed our path. We lost our way. It is where an alkaline diet will lead to improving our wellbeing.

I'm confident that you recognize the word pH relating to the acidity or alkalinity of something. Alkalinity on a scale is calculated. You should take a quick and economical home check to see where your alkalinity is and to track your alkalinity periodically.

Scientific doctors and scientists have understood this lesser-established reality for at least 70 years .... your body requires a certain pH degree or delicate equilibrium of the acid-alkaline levels in the blood to ensure the wellbeing and longevity is optimum.

Perhaps you wonder, "Why do the pH balance and alkalinity mean to me?" I know these were my thoughts when I first learned of alkaline food.

Two definitions would be used to demonstrate how acid and alkalinity are essential to the body.

1. We also realize that there is an acid in our throats. This acid is necessary for conjunction with enzymes to divide food into simple elements that can be ingested by the digestive tract. What if we have no fat in our belly? We can die of starvation in no time since the body can't use a whole slice of meat or whatever!
Can You Make Sense?

2. Various body parts need varying acidity or alkalinity amounts. The plasma, for example, needs a bit more alkaline than the stomach acids. What if you have so much acidic blood? This can nearly chew into the nerves and lungs, triggering major internal bleeding!

Although these explanations demonstrate that the various components or structures of the body need specific pH values, we should not think about this. Our question is simple because it's that we're all mostly acidic.

It is the most critical thing to remember. If the body becomes too acidic after a long period of time, it contributes to other diseases such as obesity, diabetes, lack of bone mass, high blood pressure, lung failure, and stroke. The list is infinite, as the organism eventually gives up the battle for life and falls into the state of survival as long as possible.

What's the alkaline diet like, and what would you expect?
Like other adjustments in diet or lifestyle, a phase of transition may take place. Yet if you're eating the cleanest food your body needs, you won't really have to feel thirsty, unlike other diet strategies. Plus, once you're full, you can consume all you want. You won't have to count calories, either. And you can appreciate a lot of variety, so you're never going to be bored with cooking.

Find an alkaline diet as a kind of "juice fast" for the body. It's just not that serious. You consume rich and readily digestible foods that your body longs for. Once you supply all the cells in your body that it wants so badly, the appetite goes out. Yet dull vegetables don't have to fret, as there are plenty of tasty recipes on the internet and in books.

What would you find an alternate strategy, including an alkaline diet for other eating plans?

If correctly practiced, you should assume that the fat can dissolve more quickly than for traditional plans. There are also accounts where individuals claim they drop more than two pounds a week. (And with most food plans, the weight will not be wise). When your skin becomes lighter, your vitality improves, and you would look younger.

Furthermore, the alkaline diet does two items that are essential to conventional diets.
1. It provides superior nourishment to your body's cells.
2. It naturally helps to detoxify and cleanse the cells, too.
All of these factors illustrate why an alkaline diet operates both quickly and comfortably.

The Tips for Successfully Following the Alkaline Diet

Often, stretching for the additional mile, you get to the areas you had only dreamed about. Going well on an alkaline diet will be the battle that ultimately contributes to a balanced lifestyle. An alkaline diet is an assumption that certain products, such as berries, vegetables, roots, and legumes, leave an alkaline residue or ash behind in the body. The body is strengthened by the key ingredients of rock, such as calcium, magnesium, titanium, zinc, and copper. The avoidance of asthma, malnutrition, exhaustion, and even cancer is an alkaline diet. Conscious about doing something like that?

Below are ten strategies to adopt the alkaline diet effectively.

Drink Water

Water is probably our body's most important (after oxygen) resource. Hydration in the body is very important as the water content determines the body's chemistry. Drink between 8-10 glasses of water to keep the body well hydrated (filtered to cleaned).

Avoid Acidic Drinks Like Tea, Coffee, Or Soda

Our body also attempts to regulate acid and alkaline content. There is no need to blink in carbonated drinks as the body refuses carbon dioxide as waste!

Breathe

Oxygen is the explanation that our body works, and if you provide the body with adequate oxygen, it should perform better. Sit back and enjoy two to five minutes of slow breaths. Nothing is easier than you can perform Yoga.

Avoid Food with Preservatives and Food Colors

Our body has not been programmed to absorb such substances, and the body then absorbs them or retains them as fat, and they do not damage the liver. Chemicals create acids, such that the body neutralizes them either by generating cholesterols or blanching iron from the RBCs (leading to anemia) or by extracting calcium from bones (osteoporosis).

Avoid Artificial Sweeteners

These sweeteners, which tend to be high in low fat, are potentially detrimental to the body. In addition, Saccharin, a primary ingredient in sweeteners, triggers cancer. Keep away from these things, therefore. Go for less healthy food, still a decent one.

Exercise

The alkaline and the acidic element will also be matched. This is not just a question of consuming alkaline milk. A little acid (because of muscles) often regulates natural bodywork.

Satiate Your Urges for Snack by Eating Vegetables

Whenever we are thirsty, we still consume a little fast food. Establish a tradition of consuming fresh vegetables or almonds, even walnuts.

Eat the Right Mix of Food

The fats and proteins of carbohydrates need a specific atmosphere when digested. And don't eat it all at once. Evaluate the nutritional composition and balance it accurately to create the best combination of all the nutrients you consume.

Sleep Well, Remain Calm

Seek to escape the pain. Our mind regulates the digestive system, and only when in a relaxed, focused condition can you realize it functions properly. Relax, then, and remain safe!

QUICK AND EASY ALKALINE DIET SHORTCUTS

An alkaline diet may be one of the easiest approaches to boost your mental safety and wellbeing. Some people incorrectly believe that "alkaline food" is difficult and impossible to achieve, but it's really simple to shift the diet from an unhealthy acidic diet to a balanced alkaline one. If you choose to enjoy the many health benefits of an alkaline diet, fast and simple methods to produce good results are given. You will expect improved fitness, stronger disease tolerance, and enhanced stamina by converting to an alkaline diet, among other benefits.

Add Alkaline Water to Your Diet

Drinking lots of water is important to healthy safety, so why don't alkaline water make the best of this? It's simple to make your own water at home simply by mixing a gallon of water with around half a teaspoon of baking soda. Shake and measure with a pH strip and apply additional baking soda as required to achieve a pH of 8.5 to 9. To use alkaline drops, tablets, or a jug filter both available on the market. You may also buy a water ionizer for ease to add directly to your water source. Add fresh lemon to your alkaline water before consuming a tasty and alkalizing cocktail. You may also create balanced herbal and green teas, all alkaline beverages.

Eat Plenty of Salads

Lettuce, spinach and other green leafy vegetables make huge contributions to the alkaline diet. Only add a new vegetable salad to your lunch and dinner menu and boost your wellbeing and your body. Almost all of the vegetables are alkalizing, and you can keep your salads fun and entertaining. Throughout your bowl, consider incorporating sliced cucumbers, snow peas, new green peas, and green pepper strings. By adding beans and other legumes, you can also add a touch of protein.

Eat Less Sugar

Refined sugar is very dangerous for one's safety, particularly when it promotes an acidic body reaction. If you are used to the richness of white sugar, seek to trim it down so that it can be balanced by your taste buds. White refined sugar may also be substituted with a ton of natural sugar, corn sugar, or stevia, both of which are alkalizing sweetening alternatives. However, do Nutra Sweet or High 'N Small, because they are acidifying, do not substitute sugar with chemical sweeteners. Fortunately, as you continue to use sweeteners, you can note that you enjoy a sweeter taste in your products.

Easy Food Substitutions

It is quick to create a few basic food alternatives to shift the diet from strongly acidifying to alkalizing. You eat whole grains like millet, quinoa, and wild rice instead of refined noodles and pastes. Replace the diet's red meat with nutritious shrimp, beans, and other legumes. Using good fats like olives, flaxseed, or canola oil in your cooking. You can always consume a diet high in new fruits and vegetables because the rest are alkalizing. You should sleep healthier and enjoy the safety advantages of an alkaline diet before you realize it.

DANGERS OF THE ALKALINE DIET

Alkaline Diet is becoming increasingly popular with dietitians and the health-conscious. It should not be shocking that this diet is effective in helping the body to maintain its optimum fitness, improve its strength, and attain overall wellbeing. Nevertheless, Alkaline Diet still has its share of risks, like many other diets. We give you the three greatest dangers so that you cannot fall into this diet.

1. It may not be safe to consume all alkaline food alone. The body often requires other forms and amounts of acidic substances. To remain healthy, other foods that provide the nutrients the body requires are suggested.

2. Alkalization of the diet does not fulfill the nutrients required for optimal health. Alkaline diets do not produce nutrients such as omega-3 and other main fatty acids. Of course, anyone with health awareness understands that he or she wants the nutrients of every food group except meat and dairy products. Therefore, it is important to eat foods that provide the body with acid minerals and alkaline minerals.

3. Rubber and rubber are toxic materials. If you consume water or food from a disposable bottle, you still consume toxic toxin remains or traces. That is also

valid when you consume plastic-stocked milk. That's one thing you have to recognize. The body is vulnerable with nearly all that impacts and reaches our bodies to all kinds of toxins.

Make sure the source is true when you purchase alkaline goods from the internet. It is also equally necessary to have a pH check kit to ensure that you have the right pH standard. Alkalizing the food will be pleasant if mildly completed.

CHAPTER 41

Dr Sebi Approved Food Lists and

Prohibited food

D r Sebi, in his wealth of experience as a specialist in natural health and wellness, created his specialized diets. His diets include fruits with seeds, agave syrup, wild rice, coconut oil, olive oil, and lots more. He went further to create his own fundamental six groups of food, which are; Dead, Raw, Live, Drugs, Hybrid, and Genetically Modified.

Dead Food are foods that can stay for days without going bad. These are heavily processed, synthesized, and less nutritional, some examples are fruit snacks, flavored crackers, flavored beverages, and meal replacement bars. This group of food are very common as they are fast, tasty, and convenient, but they contain chemicals, artificial colors and flavors, and unfamiliar ingredients. The consumption of such foods leads to diseases like diabetes, cancer, obesity, and heart diseases, etc.

It has been detected now that chemically processed and refined foods are significant players in the cause of body inflammation. When these dead foods accumulate in the body, it causes chronic inflammation, which results in weight gain, increased blood pressure, arthritis, and elevated blood sugar level, etc. Pains, aches, brain fog, hormonal imbalance, poor sleep are all results of the body reacting to these dead foods.

Live Food

These are foods that are either in their natural form or close to it; examples are fruits and vegetables, fish, whole grain, nuts and seeds, fish, and poultry. These foods have contrasting fortune with the dead foods as they possess antioxidants that fight inflammation and also phytochemicals. They help in the production and activation of enzymes that help produce hormones and chemical reactions in the body. These foods also boost your body defense because they possess probiotics that promote the growth of healthy bacteria that acts as the body's first response when fighting diseases.

Raw Food

Raw food, as defined by the Natural Hygiene movement in the 1800s, is any food that is cooked below a temperature lower than 115 – 118 degrees Fahrenheit. Nutrients and enzymes are assumed to be preserved when cooked in this manner and keeps food in its natural state. They are mostly vegetables, seeds, nuts, fresh fruits, and soaked legumes and grains. Consumers of raw food are usually vegan, with just a few that consume raw meat, dairy, and fish.

Experts consider raw food diets as a natural diet for humans. They say raw foods would have been our food in the wild if we had not developed agriculture, the creation of processed foods, and the domestication of animals. Some benefits of eating raw foods are improved sleep, energy, bowel movements, body fat loss, clear skin, and a clear mind, etc.

Hybrids Food

These are foods formed from the combination of two distinct fruits or vegetables. The hybrid produce is what is referred to as hybrid foods; this rarely occurs in nature but is mostly something that is engineered by men. Some examples of hybrids are seedless apples, kiwis, seedless watermelon, seedless grapes, seedless citrus fruits, and seedless persimmons. There are no real health risks in the consumption of hybrid foods.

Genetically Modified Food

Foods that are made from organisms that are genetically modified artificially are said to be genetically modified foods. This poses a significant health risk for consumers as proper work has not been done to check the production of GM foods. They are usually employed to help plant viability, but plans are on-going to alter the nutrients of foods to check allergenic potential.

Drugs

Some foods are grouped as drugs because they contain a high medicinal value, acting as a drug to the body. There are links between drugs and food, some food acts like drugs, while some drugs act as food. You should be aware of drugs that are considered as food, because they can be very harmful, unlike food servings as drugs such as green tea and coffee, they have far fewer health risks.

Approved Lists

Dr Sebi created his diets from just live and raw food groups, virtually shutting out the rest of the food groups. He encourages dieters to consume more foods that are close to a raw vegan diet, such as vegetables and fruits that are naturally grown and also whole grains. His line of thought was that the live and raw foods were electric, and they combat the acidic food waste contained in the body. Dr Sebi compiled his food list he called 'Electric Food List', he considered the best of his diets. This list continues to evolve and grow even after his demise.

For most people who eat out regularly, it is always challenging to abide by Dr Sebi's food diets. It will be great for you to start prepping yourself for vegan diet meals by learning how to prepare such meals, using olive oil, wild rice, agave syrup, etc.

Vegetable Food list

Dr Sebi strongly advocates that people should consume non-genetically modified organism foods, which includes seedless vegetables and fruits, or those modified to contain more nutrients than the natural state. He has a long, diverse list of vegetables, providing more options to make different unique meals.

These are;

- Amaranth
- Avocado
- Arame
- Bell Pepper
- Cherry and Plum Tomato
- Chayote
- Cucumber
- Dulse
- 3Dandelion Greens
- Garbanzo Beans
- Hijiki
- Izote Flower and Leaf
- Kale
- Lettuce apart from Iceberg
- Mushroom apart from Shitake

- Nori
- Nopales
- Onions
- Olives
- Okra
- Purslane Verdolaga
- Sea Vegetables
- Squash
- Tomatillo
- Turnip Greens
- Wakame
- Watercress
- Wild Arugula
- Zucchini

Fruit List

While Dr Sebi proposes a wide range of vegetables, he places a lot of restrictions on fruits. Despite this restriction, fruits have a diverse range of lists to choose from, including all varieties of berries apart from cranberries that are human-made. These are;

- Apples
- Berries
- Bananas
- Cherries
- Currants
- Cantaloupe
- Dates
- Figs
- Grapes
- Limes
- Melons
- Mango
- Orange
- Plums
- Papayas
- Prunes
- Peaches
- Pears
- Prickly Pear
- Raisins
- Sour soups
- Soft Jelly Coconut
- Tamarind

Spices and Seasoning

- Achiote
- Bay Leaf
- Basil
- Cloves
- Cayenne
- Dill
- Habanero
- Oregano
- Onion Powder
- Pure Sea Salt
- Savory
- Sweet Basil
- Sage
- Thyme
- Tarragon

Alkaline Grain

- Amaranth
- Fonio
- Kamut
- Quinoa
- Rye
- Spelt

Alkaline Sweeteners and Sugars

- 100% Pure Agave Syrup from Cactus
- Date Sugar from Dried Dates

Herbal Teas

- Burdock
- Chamomile
- Elderberry
- Fennel
- Ginger
- Red Raspberry
- Tila

Nuts and Seeds

- Brazil Nuts
- Hemp Seeds
- Raw Sesame Seeds
- Walnuts

Oils

- Avocado Oil
- Coconut Oil
- Grape seed Oil
- Hempseed Oil
- Olive Oil
- Sesame Oil

Guidelines

- Any food not listed above is not recommended.
- You should drink a gallon of water daily, preferably natural spring water.
- If you are taking pharmaceutical drugs, take Dr Sebi's product an hour prior.
- Strict adherence to Dr. Sebi's nutritional guidelines guarantees the best result in disease reversal.

- No fish, no alcohol, no animal products, no hybrid foods, and no dairy.
- Consume only the above-approved grains.
- A lot of the approved grains are sold in health food stores as bread, pasta, cereal, or flour.
- Dr Sebi's products work for 14 days within the body, as it still releases therapeutic properties.
- Do not make use of microwaves, and it kills the food.
- No consumption of seedless or canned fruits.

PROHIBITED FOODS

Foods that are not listed in the above approved Dr Sebi diet list is prohibited from being consumed, some of such foods are;

- Seedless Fruits
- Canned Fruits or Vegetables
- Fish
- Dairy
- Poultry
- Red Meat
- Fortified Foods
- Soy Products
- Wheat
- Alcohol
- Processed foods; including restaurant foods and take-outs.
- Yeast enhanced food
- Food made with baking powder
- Sugar apart from agave syrup and date sugar
- Eggs

CHAPTER 42

Breakfast Recipes

1. Banana Barley Porridge

Preparation Time: 5 minutes
Cooking Time: 30 minutes
Serving: 2
Ingredients:

- 1 cup unsweetened coconut milk, divided
- 1 small banana, peeled and sliced
- ½ cup barley

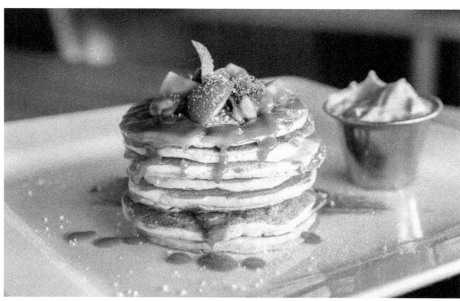

- 3 drops liquid stevia
- ¼ cup coconuts, chopped

Instructions:

1. Mix barley with half coconut milk and stevia in a bowl and mix well. Cover and refrigerate for about 6 hours.
2. Mix the barley mixture with coconut milk in a saucepan. Cook for 5 minutes on medium heat.
3. Top with chopped coconuts and banana slices. Serve.

Nutrition: Calories: 434Fat: 35gCarbs: 27gProtein: 6.7gFiber: 3.6g

2. Zucchini Muffins

Preparation Time: 10 minutes
Cooking Time: 25 minutes
Serving: 16
Ingredients:

- 1 tablespoon ground flaxseed
- 3 tablespoons water
- ¼ cup walnut butter
- 3 small-medium over-ripe bananas
- 2 small zucchinis, grated
- ½ cup coconut milk
- 1 teaspoon vanilla extract
- 2 cups coconut flour
- 1 tablespoon baking powder
- 1 teaspoon cinnamon
- ¼ teaspoon sea salt
- Optional add-ins:
- ¼ cup chocolate chips and/or walnuts

Instructions:

1. Set your oven to 375 degrees F. Grease a muffin tray with cooking spray. Mix flaxseed with water in a bowl.
2. Mash bananas in a glass bowl and stir in all the remaining ingredients. Mix well and divide the mixture into the muffin tray.
3. Bake for 25 minutes. Serve.

Nutrition: Calories: 127 Fat: 6.6g Carbs: 13gProtein: 0.7gFiber: 0.7g

---

3. Millet Porridge

Preparation Time: 10 minutes
Cooking Time: 20 minutes
Serving: 2
Ingredients:

- Pinch of sea salt
- 1 tablespoon coconuts, chopped finely
- ½ cup unsweetened coconut milk
- ½ cup millet, rinsed and drained
- 1½ cups water
- 3 drops liquid stevia

Instructions:

1. Sauté millet in a non-stick skillet for 3 minutes. Stir in salt and water. Let it boil then reduce the heat.
2. Cook for 15 minutes then stirs in remaining ingredients. Cook for another 4 minutes.
3. Serve with chopped nuts on top.

Nutrition: Calories: 219Fat: 4.5gCarbs: 38.2gProtein: 6.4gFiber: 5g

4. Jackfruit Vegetable Fry

Preparation Time: 5 minutes
Cooking Time: 5 minutes
Serving: 6
Ingredients:

- 2 small onions, finely chopped
- 2 cups cherry tomatoes, finely chopped
- 1/8 teaspoon ground turmeric
- 1 tablespoon olive oil
- 2 red bell peppers, seeded and chopped
- 3 cups firm jackfruit, seeded and chopped
- 1/8 teaspoon cayenne pepper
- 2 tablespoons fresh basil leaves, chopped
- Salt, to taste

Instructions:

1. Sauté onions and bell peppers in a greased skillet for 5 minutes. Stir in tomatoes and cook for 2 minutes.
2. Add turmeric, salt, cayenne pepper, and jackfruit. Cook for 8 minutes.
3. Garnish with basil leaves. Serve warm.

Nutrition: Calories: 236Fat: 1.8gCarbs: 48.3gProtein: 7gFiber: 0.6g

5. Zucchini Pancakes

Preparation Time: 15 minutes
Cooking Time: 8 minutes
Serving: 8
Ingredients:

- 12 tablespoons water
- 6 large zucchinis, grated
- Sea salt, to taste
- 4 tablespoons ground Flax Seeds
- 2 teaspoons olive oil
- 2 jalapeño peppers, finely chopped
- ½ cup scallions, finely chopped

Instructions:

1. Mix together water and flax seeds in a bowl and keep aside.
2. Heat oil in a large non-stick skillet on medium heat and add zucchini, salt, and black pepper.
3. Cook for about 3 minutes and transfer the zucchini into a large bowl. Stir in scallions and flax seed mixture and thoroughly mix.
4. Preheat a griddle and grease it lightly with cooking spray. Pour about ¼ of the zucchini mixture into preheated griddle and cook for about 3 minutes.
5. Flip the side carefully and cook for about 2 more minutes. Repeat with the remaining mixture in batches and serve.

Nutrition: Calories: 71Fat: 2.8gCarbs: 9.8g Protein: 3.7g   Fiber: 3.9g

6. Squash Hash

Preparation Time: 2 minutes
Cooking Time: 10 minutes
Serving: 2
Ingredients:

- 1 teaspoon onion powder
- ½ cup onion, finely chopped
- 2 cups spaghetti squash
- ½ teaspoon sea salt

Instructions:

1. Squeeze any extra moisture from spaghetti squash using paper towels. Place the squash into a bowl, then add the onion powder, onion, and salt. Stir to combine.
2. Spray a non-stick cooking skillet with cooking spray and place it over medium heat.
3. Add the spaghetti squash to pan. Cook the squash for 5 minutes, untouched. Using a spatula, flip the hash browns. Cook for an additional 5 minutes or until the desired crispness is reached. Serve and Enjoy!

Nutrition: Calories: 44Fat: 0.6gCarbs: 9.7gProtein: 0.9gFiber: 0.6g

---

7. Hemp Seed Porridge

Preparation Time: 5 minutes
Cooking Time: 5 mines
Serving: 6
Ingredients:

- 3 cups cooked hemp seed
- 1 packet Stevia
- 1 cup coconut milk

Instructions:

1. Combine the rice and coconut milk in a saucepan over medium heat for 5 minutes. Make sure to stir constantly.
2. Remove the pan from the heat and stir in the Stevia.
3. Divide among 6 bowls.
4. Serve and Enjoy!

Nutrition: Calories: 236Fat: 1.8gCarbs: 48.3gProtein: 7gFiber: 0.6g

8. Veggie Medley

Preparation Time: 5 minutes
Cooking Time: 10 minutes
Serving: 2
Ingredients:

- 1 bell pepper, any color, seeded and sliced
- Juice of ½ a lime
- 2 tablespoons fresh cilantro
- ½ teaspoon cumin
- 1 teaspoon sea salt
- 1 jalapeno, chopped
- ½ cup zucchini, sliced
- 1 cup cherry tomatoes, halved
- ½ cup mushrooms, sliced
- 1 cup broccoli florets, cooked
- 1 sweet onion, chopped

Instructions:

1. Spray a non-stick pan with cooking spray and place it over medium heat.
2. Add the onion, broccoli, bell pepper, tomatoes, zucchini, mushrooms and jalapeno. Cook for 7 minutes, or until desired doneness is reached. Stir occasionally.
3. Stir in the cumin, cilantro, and salt. Cook for 3 minutes while stirring.
4. Remove pan from heat, then add the lime juice.
5. Divide between serving plates, serve and enjoy!

Nutrition: Calories: 86 Fat: 0.07g Carbs: 17.4g Protein: 4.1g Fiber: 5.1g

9. Pumpkin Spice Quinoa

Preparation Time: 10 minutes
Cooking Time: 0 min
Serving: 2
Ingredients:

- 1 cup cooked quinoa
- 1 cup unsweetened coconut milk
- 1 large banana, mashed
- 1/4 cup pumpkin puree
- 1 teaspoon pumpkin spice
- 2 teaspoon chia seeds

Instructions:

1. Mix all the ingredients in a container.
2. Seal the lid and shake well to mix.
3. Refrigerate overnight.
4. Serve.

Nutrition: Calories: 212Fat: 11.9gCarbs: 31.7gProtein: 7.3gFiber: 2g

---

10.   Zucchini Home Fries

Preparation Time: 5 minutes
Cooking Time: 20 minutes
Serving: 2
Ingredients:

- 4 medium zucchinis
- 1 teaspoon onion powder
- 1 teaspoon sea salt
- 1 red bell pepper, seeded, diced
- ½ sweet white onion, chopped
- ¼ cup vegetable broth
- ½ cup mushrooms, sliced

Instructions:

1. In a medium-sized microwave-safe bowl, microwave the 4 zucchinis for about 4 minutes or until soft. Allow zucchinis to cool.
2. Add the broth into a large non-stick pan over medium heat, add the red bell pepper and onion. Sauté your vegetables for 5 minutes.
3. While the vegetables are cooking, slice your zucchinis into quarters.
4. Add the mushrooms, onion powder, salt and zucchinis to the pan. Cook your mixture for about 10 minutes or until the zucchinis are crisp.
5. Serve and Enjoy!

Nutrition: Calories: 337 Fat: 0.8g Carbs: 74.8gProtein: 9.3gFiber: 12.4g

11. Blackberry Pie

Preparation Time: 10 minutes
Cooking Time: 10 minutes
Serving: 4
Ingredients:

- 1 vanilla bean, cut lengthwise, deseeded
- ¼ teaspoon cinnamon
- 6 cups blackberry, sliced
- ¼ cup unsweetened coconut milk
- ½ cup orange juice, freshly squeezed

Instructions:

1. Combine all your ingredients.
2. In a medium-size skillet on medium-high heat, cook the fruit mixture. Cook the fruit mixture for 10 minutes.
3. Divide the fruit mixture among four serving dishes.
4. Top with 1 tablespoon of coconut milk.
5. Serve and Enjoy!

Nutrition: Calories: 109Fat: 0.1gCarbs: 28.5gProtein: 0.2gFiber: 4.5g

12. Figs & Ginger Fruit Compote

Preparation Time: 10 minutes
Cooking Time: 10 minutes
Serving: 4
Ingredients:

- 1 apple, peeled, cored and diced
- 2 tangerines, peeled and sectioned
- ½ cup plums, dried and halved
- ½ cup figs, stemmed and quartered
- 1 packet Stevia
- ½ teaspoon cloves
- ½ teaspoon cinnamon
- 1 teaspoon ginger, fresh and grated
- 1 vanilla bean, split lengthwise, deseeded
- ¼ cup dark cherries
- 1 cup of filtered water

Instructions:

1. In a saucepan, mix all of the ingredients.
2. Bring to a simmer over medium heat and cook for 10 minutes, stirring occasionally or until the fruit is tender.
3. Remove from the heat source, then let stand for 30 minutes.
4. Serve warm and Enjoy!

Nutrition: Calories: 102 Fat: 0.4g Carbs: 26g Protein: 1g Fiber: 4.2g

---

13.   Lime & Mint Summer Fruit Salad

Preparation Time: 10 minutes
Cooking Time: 0 minutes
Serving: 4
Ingredients:

- ¼ cup apple, peeled and diced
- ¼ cup grapes
- 2 tablespoons mint, fresh and chopped
- 2 tablespoons Seville orange juice, freshly squeezed
- ¼ cup strawberries
- ¼ cup peaches, peeled and diced
- ¼ cup tangerine slices
- ¼ cup cantaloupe, small bite-size pieces
- ¼ cup honeydew melon, small bite-size pieces
- ¼ cup watermelon, small bite-size pieces

Instructions:

1. In a mixing bowl, combine all of the fruit.
2. Add the Seville orange juice, mint and mix well.
3. Serve chilled and enjoy!

Nutrition: Calories: 32 Fat: 0.02g Carbs: 7.8g Protein: 0.6g Fiber: 0.09g

14.   Dr. Sebi Granola

Preparation Time: 2 minutes
Cooking Time: 15 minutes
Serving: 4
Ingredients:

- 1 cup slivered coconuts
- 1 cup flaked unsweetened coconut
- ½ cup raisins
- ½ cup flaxseed
- ½ teaspoon nutmeg
- ½ teaspoon cinnamon
- ¼ teaspoon ginger
- ¼ teaspoon sea salt
- ½ cup unsweetened dried pineapple pieces
- ¼ cup coconut oil

Instructions:

1.Preheat your oven to 350° Fahrenheit.
2.In a bowl, combine the coconut, flaxseed, coconuts, raisins, ginger, cinnamon, nutmeg, vanilla bean seeds, salt, and coconut oil. Mix until well combined.
3.Spread the mix on a baking sheet and bake for 15 minutes, occasionally stirring, until golden brown.
4.Remove from your oven and cool, without stirring.
5.Once cooled, stir in the pineapple pieces.
6.Store in an airtight container.

Nutrition: Calories: 210Fat: 8gCarbs: 29gProtein: 6gFiber: 4g

15. Vegetable Pancakes

Preparation Time: 5 minutes
Cooking Time: 5 minutes
Serving: 2
Ingredients:

- ½ white onion, grated
- 1 yellow squash, roughly chopped
- 1 zucchini, peeled and chopped
- 1 zucchini, roughly chopped
- ½ teaspoon onion powder
- ¼ cup filtered water, as needed
- 1 teaspoon salt
- ¼ cup coconut flour
- 4 scallions

Instructions:

1. Add the yellow squash, zucchini, zucchini, scallions, coconut flour, onion, salt, and onion powder in a food processor. Pulse until blended.
2. Add the water to the mixture to make moist but not runny. The batter will be thick.
3. Spray Pan with cooking spray and heat over medium high heat.
4. Using an ice-cream scoop to drop batter into pan. Use a fork to spread your mixture evenly over pan, pressing down on the pancakes. Brown on both sides of pancakes, cooking for about 5 minutes total.
5. Serve hot and Enjoy!

Nutrition: Calories: 254Fat: 12.1gCarbs: 33.4gProtein: 6.3gFiber: 7.2g

16.   Turnip Bowl

Preparation Time: 5 minutes
Cooking Time: 10 minutes
Serving: 2
Ingredients:

- 2 turnips, peeled and cubed
- 1 tablespoon coconut oil
- 1 red bell pepper, seeded and chopped
- 1 sweet onion, chopped
- ¼ cup mushrooms, sliced
- 4 cups kale
- 2 chive stalks, chopped
- 1 teaspoon onion powder
- 1 teaspoon onion powder
- ½ teaspoon sea salt
- ½ teaspoon Bouquet Garn herb blended, or other dried herbs like sage or rosemary

Instructions:

1.In a bowl, combine the turnips, red bell pepper, mushrooms, kale, chives, onion, oil, onion powder, and onion powder.
2.Heat a non-stick cooking pan over medium heat, and cook the vegetables, stirring often for about 10 minutes, or until tender.
3.Serve and Enjoy!

Nutrition: Calories: 181Fat: 1.5gCarbs: 37.8gProtein: 5.6gFiber: 8.1g

17.   Hempseed Milk

Preparation Time: 10 minutes
Cooking Time: 5 minutes
Serving: 6
Ingredients:

- 2 tbsp. Hemp Seeds
- 2 cups Spring Water
- 1/8 tsp. Sea Salt
- 2 tbsp. Agave
- 1 cup Strawberries (Optional)

Instructions:

1.Mash all the ingredients except the fruits into the blender.
2.Allow them to blend for 2 minutes.

3.Add fruits to the milk and allow it to blend for an added 30 seconds.

4.Store the milk in the refrigerator until its cold.

5.Afterwards, serve and enjoy your Hemp Milk!

Nutrition: Calories: 43Fat: 1.6gCarbs: 9.7gProtein: 0.1gFiber: 0.6g

---

18.　　Apple Pie Recipe

Preparation Time: 11 minutes
Cooking Time: 5 minutes
Serving: 1
Ingredients:

- 3-4 lbs. baking Apples
- 1/2 cup Agave
- 1/2 cup Date Sugar
- 1/2 tsp. Sea Salt / 1 tsp. Sea Salt
- 1/4 tsp. Ground Cloves
- 1 tsp. Allspice
- 2 cups Spelt Flour
- 1/3 cup Grape seed Oil
- 1/2 cup Spring Water
- Limes (optional)

Tools:

- Apple Slicer/Corer
- Vegetable Peeler
- Food Processor (optional)
- Pizza Cutter

Instructions

1.Preheat your oven to 425°F while cutting the apples into thin slices.

2.Place allspice, gloves, date sugar, apples and half teaspoon of sea salt to a skillet.

3.Set your cooker to low heat. Mix the ingredients and simmer for 20 minutes.

4.Place spelt flour and a tablespoon of sea salt to a processor and blend for 10 seconds.

5.Carefully add grape seed oil while mixing. Add spring water to form a ball.

6. Place the dough into a pie pan for removal of excess.

7.Add agave or any other insufficient ingredient to the apple mixture.

8.With a knife or pizza cutter, cut out 1-inch strips from the other half of dough.

9.Lay the strips vertically and horizontally on the pie.

10. Bake in the oven until it is golden brown.

Nutrition: Calories: 42Fat: 1.8gCarbs: 9.7gProtein: 0.1gFiber: 0.6g

19.   Donuts Recipe

Preparation Time: 10 minutes
Cooking Time: 3 minutes
Serving: 1
Ingredients:

- 3/4 cup Garbanzo Bean Flour (Chickpea Flour)
- 1/4 cup Sparkling Spring Water
- 1 tsp. Sea Moss Gel
- 1/2 tsp. Sea Salt
- •1/4 tsp. Ground Cloves
- Grape Seed Oil
- Coconut Flakes (optional)
- Glaze (Mix coconut oil and agave together to your taste) (optional)

Tools:

Donut Pan

Instructions:

1. With the exception of grape seed oil, add the other ingredients into a large bowl. Mix till it is well blended.
2. Preheat your donut pan to 350°F then sprinkle oil.
3. Turn the batter into the donut pan and bake for 14 minutes.
4. set aside the donuts until they are cool. Cut out the centers afterward.
5. Adorn the top with coconut flakes and glaze.

Nutrition: Calories: 41Fat: 1.6gCarbs: 9.7gProtein: 0.1gFiber: 0.6g

20.   Pizza Crust

Preparation Time: 10 minutes
Cooking Time: 3 minutes
Serving: 6
Ingredients:

- 1 1/2 cups Spelt Flour
- 1 tsp. Onion po wder
- 1 tsp. Oregano
- 2 tsp. Sesame seeds
- 1 tsp. Sea Salt
- 2 tsp. Agave
- 2 tsp. Grape seed Oil
- 1 cup Spring Water

Instructions:

1.Preheat your oven to 400°F.

2.Mix all your ingredients in a medium-sized bowl alongside half cup of spring water.

3.Add water and flour to make a ball.

4.Sprinkle your baking sheet with grape seed oil then roll out the donuts on it.

5.Poke holes in the crust with a fork, sprinkle grape seed oil on it then bake for 15 minutes.

6.While the crust is baking, prepare either a tomato or avocado sauce.

7.Once the crust is ready, add onions, peppers, mushrooms, and Brazil nuts cheese and pizza sauce. Then, bake the pizza for 20 minutes.

Nutrition: Calories: 49Fat: 1.9gCarbs: 9.7gProtein: 0.1gFiber: 0.6g

21.   Dr. Sebi Hot Sauce Recipe

Preparation Time: 10 minutes
Cooking Time: 5 minutes
Ingredients:

- 3 Habaneros
- 1/3 cup spring water
- 1/4 cup Red Pepper
- 1/4 cup Onions, diced

- 1/2 teaspoon Sea Salt
- 1 tablespoon Onion Powder
- 2 tablespoons Lime Juice
- 1 tablespoon Grape Seed Oil

Tools:

- Blender
- Strainer

Pro Tip: Remember to cook habaneros whole and maintain proper ventilation as these peppers are powerful.

Instructions:

1.Set your cooker to medium heat. The, Sprinkle grape seed oil on your skillet.

2.Sautee sea salt, peppers, habaneros and onions for 4 minutes.

3.Separate the stems from the habaneros then include vegetable and all other ingredients to the blender.

4.Blend the sauce until the seeds are all out and the sauce is smooth.

5.Your Hot Sauce Recipe is ready to be dished.

Nutrition: Calories: 40Fat: 1.9gCarbs: 9.7gProtein: 0.1gFiber: 0.6g

CHAPTER 43

Lunch Recipes

22.   Cheesy Spinach Bake

Preparation Time: 10 Minutes

Cooking Time: 40 Minutes

Servings: 4

Ingredients:

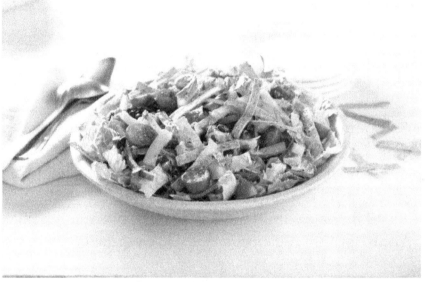

- Nonstick cooking spray
- 2 tablespoons grass-fed butter
- 2 cups chopped onion
- 2 garlic cloves, minced
- 2 zucchinis, chopped into bite-size pieces
- 2 cups fresh spinach
- 3 eggs, beaten
- ¼ cup heavy (whipping) cream
- ½ teaspoon salt
- ¼ teaspoon freshly ground black pepper
- 1½ cups shredded mozzarella cheese
- ½ cup grated Parmesan cheese

Instructions:

1. Preheat the oven to 350°F. Coat a 9-inch glass pie plate with cooking spray.

2. In a skillet over medium-high heat, melt the butter. Add the onion and garlic and sauté for 2 minutes.

3. Add the zucchini and cook for another 4 minutes. Add the spinach and stir until wilted. Transfer the mixture and spread it evenly with a spatula.

4. In a small bowl, mix together the eggs, cream, salt, and pepper. Pour the mixture over the vegetables.

5. Top with the mozzarella and Parmesan cheeses and bake for 30 to 35 minutes. Serve warm.

Nutrition: Calories: 386 Cal Fat: 30 g Protein: 21 g Carbs: 8g Fiber: 2g

23.   Fakeachini Alfredo

Preparation Time: 15 Minutes
Cooking Time: 5 Minutes
Servings: 1
Ingredients:

- ½ tablespoon extra-virgin olive oil
- 1 teaspoon minced garlic
- ¼ teaspoon salt
- ¼ teaspoon garlic powder
- 1 wedge Laughing Cow Swiss cheese, cubed
- 1 to 2 tablespoons heavy (whipping) cream
- 3 tablespoons grated Parmesan cheese
- 2 ounces seitan strips or cubes
- ⅓ Cup cooked spaghetti squash
- 1 tablespoon chopped fresh parsley

Instructions:

1. Warm the olive oil. Add the garlic, salt, and garlic powder and stir for 1 to 2 minutes or until fragrant.

2. Add the cheese and stir until melted. Thin the sauce to your desired consistency with the cream. Continue to stir until melted.

3. Add the seitan to the sauce.

4. Place the squash in a serving bowl, pour the sauce on top, and sprinkle with the parsley.

Nutrition: Calories: 452 Cal Fat: 24 g Protein: 52 g Carbs: 7 g Fiber: 3 g

24. Cheesy Cauliflower Mac 'N' Cheese

Preparation Time: 10 Minutes
Cooking Time: 30 Minutes
Serving: 6
Ingredients:

- Nonstick cooking spray
- 1 cauliflower head, chopped into small florets
- 8 ounces heavy (whipping) cream
- 4 ounces shredded sharp cheddar cheese
- 4 ounces grated Parmesan cheese
- 2 ounces cream cheese
- 1 teaspoon salt
- ¼ teaspoon freshly ground black pepper

Instructions:

1. Preheat the oven to 375°F. Spray an 8-by-8-inch baking dish with cooking spray.

2. Place the cauliflower in a microwave-safe bowl and cook for 3 minutes on high. Drain any excess liquid.

3. Combine the heavy cream, cheddar cheese, Parmesan cheese, cream cheese, salt, and pepper.

4. Pour the cheese sauce over the cauliflower and toss to coat.

Nutrition: Calories: 324 Fat: 28g Protein: 13g Carbs: 5g Fiber: 1g

25. Alkaline Flatbread

Preparation Time: 5 minutes
Cooking Time: 30 minutes
Serving: 5
Ingredients:

- 2 cups Spelt Flour
- 2 tbsps. Grape seed Oil
- 3/4 cup Clean Water
- 1 tbsp. Sea Salt
- 2 tsps. Oregano
- 2 tsps. Basil
- 2 tsps. Onion Powder
- 1/4 tsp. Cayenne

Instructions:

1. Mix together the flour and the seasonings until properly blended.
2. Add in the oil and 1/2 cup of the clean water into the mix.
3. Add in flour to the workspace and knead the dough for about five minutes, then divide the dough into 6 equal portions.
4. Roll out each ball into 4-inch circles.
5. Place an un-greased skillet on moderate heat.
6. Cook the rolled balls as you flip them after every 3 minutes until done.
7. Enjoy.

Nutrition: Calories: 107 kcal; Fat: 3.9g; Carbs: 1.5g; Protein: 0.001g

---

26.   Lunch Salad

Preparation Time: 11 minutes
Cooking Time: 15 Minutes
Serving: 2
Ingredients

- 1/2 seeded cucumber
- 2 cups watercress
- 2 tbsp. olive oil
- 1 tbsp. key lime juice
- Salt and cayenne pepper, to taste.

Instructions

1. Mix the key lime and olive oil until meticulously combined.
2. Arrange cucumber and watercress.
3. Add the dressing and dust with pepper and salt, to your taste.

Nutrition: Calories: 251 Fat: 3.8g Carbs: 54g Protein: 6.5g Fiber: 3.5g

27.   Margherita Pizza

Preparation Time: 10 Minutes
Cooking Time: 5 Minutes
Servings: 1
Ingredients:

- 1 tablespoon psyllium husk powder
- ½ teaspoon dried oregano
- 2 large eggs
- 1 tablespoon avocado oil
- 3 tablespoons low-sugar marinara sauce
- 2 tablespoons grated Parmesan cheese
- ½ cup sliced mozzarella cheese
- 1 tablespoon chopped fresh basil

Instructions:

1. Line a baking sheet with aluminum foil. Turn the oven to low broil. Combine the psyllium husk powder, salt, oregano, and eggs in a blender. Blend for 30 seconds. Set aside.
2. In a sauté pan or skillet, over high heat, warm the avocado oil. Pour the crust mixture into the pan, spreading it out into a circle.
3. Cook until the edges and then flip the crust and cook for an additional minute.
4. Transfer the crust to the baking sheet. Spread the marinara sauce over the top and cover with the Parmesan and mozzarella cheeses.
5. Broil until the cheese is melted
6. Top with the basil and enjoy.

Nutrition: Calories: 545 Cal Fat: 41 g Protein: 32 g Carbs: 12 g Fiber: 8 g

28.   Creamy Onion Soup

Preparation Time: 10minutes
Cooking Time: 65 Minutes
Servings: 4
Ingredients:

- 3 tbsp. olive oil
- 3 cups thinly sliced white onions
- 2 garlic cloves, thinly sliced
- 2 tsp. almond flour
- ½ cup dry white wine
- Salt and black pepper to taste
- 2 sprigs chopped thyme
- 2 cups hot vegetable broth
- 2 cups almond milk
- 1 cup grates Swiss cheese

Instructions:

1. Heat the olive oil in a pot. Sauté the onions for 10 minutes or until softened, stirring regularly to avoid browning. Reduce the heat and cook for 15 minutes while occasionally stirring.

2. Mix in the garlic, cook further for 10 minutes or until the onions caramelize.

3. Stir in the almond flour well, wine, and increase the heat. Season with salt, black pepper, thyme, and pour in the hot vegetable broth.

4. Pour in the almond milk and half of the Swiss cheese. Stir until the cheese melts, adjust the taste with salt, black pepper, and dish the soup.

Nutrition: Calories: 183 Cal Fat: 14.7 g Carbs: 8 g Fiber: 2 g Protein: 8 g

---

29.   Alkaline-Electric Ice Cream

Preparation Time: 15 minutes
Cooking Time: 25 Minutes
Serving: 2
Ingredients:

- Agave syrup
- 3 tablespoons of homemade walnut milk
- 2 ripe mangoes
- 2 burro bananas

Instructions:

1. Peel and then cut all your mangoes into small cubes.

2. Peel and slice the burro bananas.

3. Put both the banana mango and pieces in a baking sheet lined with parchment paper and freeze.

4. Place your frozen fruit in a food processor and add the sweetener and the homemade walnut milk.

5.Blend for 4 minutes.

6.You need to stop it throughout to push it down and stir it around.

7.Serve and enjoy.

Nutrition: Calories: 22.1Fat: 3.7gCarbs: 54gProtein: 5.5g Fiber: 3.5g

---

30.   Basil Zucchinis and Eggplants

Preparation Time: 10 Minutes
Cooking Time: 20 Minutes
Servings: 4
Ingredients:

- 1 tablespoon olive oil
- 2 zucchinis, sliced
- 1 eggplant, roughly cubed
- 2 scallions, chopped
- 1 tablespoon sweet paprika
- Juice of 1 lime
- 1 teaspoon fennel seeds, crushed
- Salt and black pepper to the taste
- 1 tablespoon basil, chopped

Instructions:

1. Heat up a pan with the oil and add scallions and fennel seeds and sauté for 5 minutes.

2. Add zucchinis, eggplant and the other ingredients, toss, cook over medium heat for 15 minutes more.

Nutrition: Calories: 97 Cal Fat: 4 g Fiber: 2 g Carbs: 6 g Protein: 2 g

---

31.   Nori~burritos

Preparation Time: 11 minutes
Cooking Time: 15 Minutes
Serving: 2

Ingredients:

- A handful of sprouted hemp seeds
- 1/2 mango, ripe
- A handful of amaranths
- 1 tbs. tahini
- Sesame seeds, to taste
- 450 gr. cucumber
- 4 sheets nori seaweed
- 1 zucchini, small
- 1 avocado, ripe

Instructions:

1.Place the Nori sheet on board with the sparkling side facing down.

2.Arrange all the ingredients on the nori sheet, leaving a margin of an inch uncovered with the nori to the right.

3.Fold the sheet of nori from the edge close to you up and over the fillings.

4.Sprinkle with sesame seeds when you cut in thick slices.

Nutrition: Calories: 271 Fat: 3.7g Carbs: 54g Protein: 6.5g Fiber: 3.5g

---

32.   Detox Smoothie for lunch

Preparation Time: 11 minutes

Cooking Time: 15 Minutes

Serving: 2

Ingredients

- 2 tbsp. key lime juice
- 1/2 cup ginger tea
- 1/2 burro banana
- 1/2 cup soft jelly coconut water
- 1 cup Romaine lettuce
- 1/4 cup blueberries

Instructions

1.Prepare the tea and cool

2.Blend all ingredients

3.Serve and enjoy!

Nutrition: Calories: 271Fat: 3.7gCarbs: 54gProtein: 6.5g Fiber: 3.5g

33.   Berry Sorbet for lunch

Preparation Time: 11 minutes
Cooking Time: 15 Minutes
Serving: 2
Ingredients

- 1-1/2 tsp. spelt
- 1/2 cup date sugar
- 2 cups water
- Flour
- 2 cups strawberries

Instructions

1. In a large saucepan, dissolve the flour and date sugar in the water over low heat
2. Boil for ten minutes.
3. When the syrup is cooled, add the squashed fruit and mix well.
4. Cut the sorbet into small portions, and then process in a blender until creamy and smooth.
5. Put in plastic and freeze open until it is rock-hard.
6. Put the sorbet into the freezer again and allow it to freeze for an extra 3 hours.

Nutrition: Calories: 271Fat: 3.7gCarbs: 54gProtein: 5.5g Fiber: 3.5g

34.   Chickpea Burger

Preparation Time: 5 minutes
Cooking Time: 10 minutes
Serving: 3
Ingredients:

- 1 cup Garbanzo Bean Flour
- 1/2 cup diced Onions
- 1/2 cup diced Green Peppers
- 1/2 cup diced Kale
- 1 diced Plum Tomato
- 2 tsps. Oregano
- 2 tsps. Onion Powder
- 2 tsps. Sea Salt
- 1/2 tsp. Ginger Powder
- 1/2 tsp. Cayenne Powder
- 1/2 cup Clean Water

Instructions:

1.Mix all the vegetables and seasonings together then mix them in flour.

2.Slowly add drinking water and mix properly until the mixture could be formed right into a patty.

3.In a skillet, pour oil and cook the patties on moderate heat for 3 minutes on both sides as you continue flipping until the sides are brown.

4.Serve on alkaline flatbread.

5.Serve.

Nutrition: Calories: 272 kcal; Carbs: 39g; Fat: 9g; Proteins: 7g

CHAPTER 44

Dinner Recipes

35.   Strawberry Daiquiri

Preparation Time: 10 Minutes
Cooking Time: 24 Minutes
Servings: 4
Ingredients

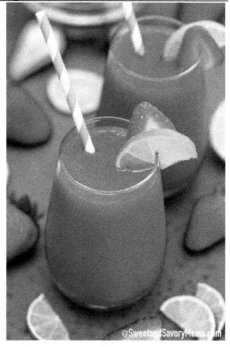

- 1 (10 ounce) can froze strawberry daiquiri concentrate
- 1 (10 ounce) can froze strawberry daiquiri concentrate
- 1 1/2 cups frozen strawberries
- 1 cup ice cube

Instructions

1. Combine all ingredients in blender until all the ice is crushed.
2. Add more ice-cubes for the right texture.

Nutrition: Calories: 113 Cal Fat: 21.3 g Carbs: 5 g Fiber: 2 g, Protein: 4 g

36. Diabetic Virgin White Sangria

Preparation Time: 5 Minutes
Cooking Time: 4 Minutes
Servings: 1
Ingredients

- 4 cups ocean spray white cranberry juice with Splenda
- 2 cups fresh fruit, sliced
- 1 cup diet lemon-lime soda
- 1 lime, juice of

Instructions

1. Combine ingredients except the soda in a large pitcher and chill for at least 1 hour.
2. When serving, add the soda. Serve with a pretty fruit garnish.

Nutrition: Calories: 126 Cal Fat: 21.3 g Carbs: 5 g Fiber: 2 g, Protein: 4 g

37. Wow Cola Chicken

Preparation Time: 15 Minutes
Cooking Time: 14 Minutes
Servings: 1
Ingredients

- 16 ounces boneless chicken breasts
- 1 (12 ounce) can diet cola
- 1 cup ketchup

Instructions

1. Place chicken in crockpot and then top with ketchup and then pour cola over all.
2. Cook on low for 6-8 hours.

Nutrition
Calories: 306 Cal Fat: 21.3 g Carbs: 5 g Fiber: 2 g, Protein: 4 g

38.   Yummy Berry Cooler

Preparation Time: 5 Minutes
Cooking Time: 4 Minutes
Servings: 1
Ingredients

- 2 2/3 cups cranberry~raspberry juice (I use the Splenda sweetened light version)
- 1 cup diet lemon~lime soda
- Cool Whip
- 4 cherries

Instructions

1. Combine first 3 ingredients.
2. Add ice if desired.

Nutrition: Calories: 106 Cal Fat: 21.3 g Carbs: 3 g Fiber: 1 g, Protein: 4 g

39.   Warm Apple Delight

Preparation Time: 5 Minutes
Cooking Time: 4 Minutes
Servings: 1
Ingredients

- 2 red apples, cored & cut in half
- 1 (375 ml) canflavoured diet cola (cherry or strawberry suggested)
- 1 pinch Splenda sugar substitute or 1 pinch Equal sugar substitute
- 1 pinch cinnamon

Instructions

1. Place the Apple in a baking dish, skin side down and pour the cola over.
2. Sprinkle with sweetener & cinnamon.
3. Bake in a pre~heated oven at 180.C for 25~30 minutes.

Nutrition: Calories: 156 Cal Fat: 21.3 g Carbs: 5 g Fiber: 2 g, Protein: 4 g

40. Low Carb Sweet and Sour Chicken

Preparation Time: 15 Minutes
Cooking Time: 4 Minutes
Servings: 2
Ingredients

- 1 ~1 1/2 lb. boneless chicken, cut up
- 1 cup white onion (you can leave the chunks big so you can pick them out)
- 12 ounces diet orange soda (Diet Rite Tangerine works great)
- 2 tablespoons soy sauce
- 2 tablespoons white vinegar
- 1 teaspoon ground ginger
- 1/2 teaspoon garlic powder
- 1/4 teaspoon cayenne pepper
- Black pepper, to taste

Instructions

1. Brown chicken and onions in a non-stick pan sprayed with cooking spray.
2. When chicken is brown, add the remaining ingredients.
3. Cover and simmer for about 20 minutes until the chicken is tender and thoroughly cooked.
4. Uncover and reduce liquid until it makes a syrupy sauce.
5. A little arrowroot powder may be added to thicken the sauce, if desired.

Nutrition: Calories: 106 Cal Fat: 21.3 g Carbs: 5 g Fiber: 2 g, Protein: 8 g

41. Orange Dream Cake

Preparation Time: 5 Minutes
Cooking Time: 4 Minutes
Servings: 1
Ingredients

- 18 1/4 ounces orange cake mix
- 10 fluid ounces diet orange soda
- 2 egg whites

CEILING

- 3 1/2 ounces fat-free, sugar-free vanilla pudding mix
- 1 cup of skim milk

- 6 ounces unsweetened orange gelatin, divided (2 packets)
- 1 cup of hot water
- 1 cup of cold water

- 1 teaspoon vanilla extract
- 8 oz Cool Whip Free, thawed

Instructions:

1. Mix the sponge cake mixture, the soda and the egg white.
2. Pour into 9 x 13-inch baking pan.
3. Bake according to the instructions on the box.
4. Use a meat fork to poke holes in the top of the entire pie.
5. Let cake cool.
6. In a medium bowl, mix 1 box of orange gelatin, 1 cup of hot water, and 1 cup of cold water.
7. Pour the gelatin mixture over the cake.
8. Refrigerate for 2 to 3 hours.
9. Meanwhile, mix remaining gelatin box, vanilla pudding mix, skim milk, and vanilla. Hit well.
10. Add the whipped glaze to this mixture and spread it over the cake.
11. Refrigerate until serving.

Nutrition: Calories: 106 Cal Fat: 11.3 g Carbs: 5 g Fiber: 2 g, Protein: 9 g

42.   Capriosa De Fresca

Preparation Time: 5 Minutes
Cooking Time: 7 Minutes
Servings: 1
Ingredients

- 1 1/2 ounces strawberry vodka (Stoli, Smirnoff, etc)
- 1 teaspoon sugar
- 7 ounces diet 7-Up
- 3 fresh strawberries, sliced
- 2 slices limes (small wedges)

Instructions

1. Place the strawberries, lime wedges in the bottom of your cocktail glass. Muddle.

2. Add the strawberry vodka and 7-Up.

3. Gradually add the sugar (You can also add the sugar in the first step, this will make the fruit a little sweeter.

Nutrition: Calories: 216 Cal Fat: 21.3 g Carbs: 5 g Fiber: 2 g, Protein: 6 g

43.   Delicious Low-Cal Smoothie

Preparation Time: 5 Minutes
Cooking Time: 4 Minutes
Servings: 1
Ingredients

- 1 cup frozen raspberries
- 1 1/2 cups frozen strawberries
- 1 cup pineapple
- 355 ml diet Sprite

Instructions

1. If your pineapple isn't already chopped up, chop it into pieces so it's easier to blend.

2. Add all fruits into a blender.

3. Add the can of sprite, add less than the whole can if you want a thicker smoothie.

4. Blend on high power until smooth.

5. Serve in your favorite glasses, either with spoons or straws.

Nutrition: Calories: 126 Cal Fat: 21.3 g Carbs: 5 g Fiber: 2 g, Protein: 4 g

---

44.   Diabetic Mock Sangria

Preparation Time: 5 Minutes
Cooking Time: 4 Minutes
Servings: 1
Ingredients

- 2 cups orange juice, ice cold
- 1 cup unsweetened white grape juice, cold
- 1 cup low calorie cranberry juice cocktail
- 1 bottle (1 liter) lemon-lime diet soda, chilled ice cube
- 2 cups fresh fruit, oranges, sliced, thinly sliced, and halved or 2 cups lemons or 2 cups lemon or 2 cups pineapple chunks
- Sprig of fresh mint

Instructions

1. In a large bowl or jar, mix chilled orange juice, white grape juice, and cranberry juice.
2. Add lemon-lime drink; stir gently.
3. Fill each of the 10 glasses with about two-thirds of the ice.
4. Divide the fruit among the cups.
5. Pour the juice mixture into glasses and stir gently.

Nutrition: Calories: 106 Cal Fat: 21.3 g Carbs: 5 g Fiber: 2 g, Protein: 4 g

---

45.   Berries Salad with Whipped Ricotta Cream

Preparation Time: 5 Minutes
Cooking Time: 4 Minutes
Servings: 1

Ingredients

- 2 cups strawberries, freshly sliced
- 1 cup blueberries
- 1/4 cup diet lemon-lime soda, divided
- 1 tablespoon fresh mint leaves, chopped
- 1/2 cup skim milk ricotta cheese
- 2 1/2 teaspoons lemon zest
- 2 tablespoons nonfat sour cream

Instructions

1. Toss strawberries, blueberries, two tablespoons of soda, and mint together in a medium bowl; set aside for 10 minutes.

2. Meanwhile, combine ricotta, remaining two tablespoons of soda, and lemon zest in another bowl.

3. Beat with a hand mixer until light and fluffy; Add the cream.

4. Place about 3/4 cup of the berry mixture and top each serving with 1/3 cup of sour cream.

Nutrition: Calories: 119 Cal Fat: 11.3 g Carbs: 5 g Fiber: 2 g, Protein: 4 g

---

46.   Seitan Tex-Mex Casserole

Preparation Time: 5 Minutes
Cooking Time: 35 Minutes
Servings: 4
Ingredients:

- 2 tbsp. vegan butter
- 1 ½ lb. seitan
- 3 tbsp. Tex-Mex seasoning
- 2 tbsp. chopped jalapeño peppers
- ½ cup crushed tomatoes
- Salt and black pepper to taste
- ½ cup shredded vegan cheese
- 1 tbsp. chopped fresh green onion to garnish
- 1 cup sour cream for serving

Instructions:

1. Melt the vegan butter in a medium skillet over medium heat and cook the seitan until brown, 10 minutes.

3. Stir in the Tex-Mex seasoning, jalapeño peppers, and tomatoes; simmer for 5 minutes and adjust the taste with salt and black pepper.
4. Transfer and level the mixture in the baking dish. Top with the vegan cheese and bake in the upper rack of the oven for or
5. Remove the dish and garnish with the green onion.
6. Serve the casserole with sour cream.

Nutrition: Calories: 464 Cal Fat: 37.8 g Carbs: 12 g Fiber: 2 g Protein: 24 g

47.   Mushroom, Spinach and Turmeric Frittata

Preparation Time: 10 minutes
Cooking Time: 40 minutes
Servings: 6
Ingredients:

- ½ tsp. pepper
- ½ tsp. salt
- 1 tsp. turmeric
- 5-oz firm tofu
- 4 large eggs
- 6 large egg whites
- ¼ cup water
- 1 lb. fresh spinach
- 6 cloves freshly chopped garlic
- 1 large onion, chopped
- 1 lb. button mushrooms, sliced

Instructions:
1. Grease a 10-inch nonstick and ovenproof skillet and preheat oven to 350oF.
2. Place skillet on medium-high fire and add mushrooms. Cook until golden brown.
4. Add garlic, sauté for 30 seconds.
5. Add water and spinach, cook, while covered until spinach is wilted, around 2 minutes.
6. In a blender, puree pepper, salt, turmeric, tofu, eggs, and egg whites until smooth. Pour into skillet once the liquid is fully evaporated.
8. Pop skillet into oven and bake until the center is set around 25-30 minutes.

9. Remove the skillet from the oven and let it stand for ten minutes before inverting and transferring to a serving plate.
10. Cut into six equal wedges, serve and enjoy.

Nutrition: Calories 358 Fat 6g Carbs 65g Protein 21g Fiber 12g

---

48.　　Roasted Root Vegetables

Preparation Time: 10 minutes
Cooking time: 1 hour and 30 minutes
Servings: 6
Ingredients:

- 2 tbsp. olive oil
- 1 head garlic, cloves separated and peeled
- 1 large turnip, peeled and cut into ½-inch pieces
- 1 medium-sized red onion, cut into ½-inch pieces
- 1 ½ lbs. beets, trimmed but not peeled, scrubbed and cut into ½-inch pieces
- 1 ½ lbs. Yukon gold potatoes, unpeeled, cut into ½-inch pieces
- 2 ½ lbs. butternut squash, peeled, seeded, cut into ½-inch pieces

Instructions:
Grease 2 rimmed and large baking sheets. Preheat oven to 425oF.
Mix all ingredients thoroughly.
Into the two baking sheets, evenly divide the root vegetables, spread in one layer.
Season generously with pepper and salt.
Pop into the oven and roast until golden brown and tender.
Remove from the oven for at least 15 minutes before serving.

Nutrition: Calories 278 Fat 5g Carbs 57g Protein 6g Fiber 10g

49.   Tropical Fruit Parfait

Preparation Time: 10 minutes
Cooking Time: 10 minutes
Servings: 1
Ingredients:

- 1 tbsp. toasted sliced almonds
- ¼ cup plain soy yogurt
- ½ cup of fruit combination cut into ½-inch cubes (pineapple, mango and kiwi)

Instructions:

Prepare fresh fruit by peeling and slicing into ½-inch cubes.
Place cubed fruit in a bowl and top with a dollop of soy yogurt.
Garnish with sliced almonds and if desired, refrigerate for an hour before serving.

Nutrition: Calories 119 Fat 2g Carbs 25g Protein 2g Fiber 1g

50.   Cinnamon Chips with Avocado-Strawberry Salsa

Preparation Time: 10 minutes
Cooking Time: 10 minutes
Servings: 6
Ingredients:

- 3/8 tsp. salt
- 2 tsp. fresh lime juice
- 1 tsp. minced seeded jalapeno pepper
- 2 tbsp. minced fresh cilantro
- 1 cup finely chopped strawberries
- 1 ½ cups finely chopped, peeled and ripe avocado
- ½ tsp. ground cinnamon
- 2 tsp. sugar
- 6 6-inch brown rice tortillas
- 2 tsp. olive oil

Instructions:

1. Preheat oven to 350oF.
2. Prepare the cinnamon chips by brushing olive oil all over the brown rice tortilla.
3. Mix together cinnamon and sugar.

4. Sprinkle cinnamon-sugar mixture evenly all over each of the brown rice tortilla.

5. Cut up each tortilla into 12 wedges, evenly and place on a baking sheet. If needed you can bake tortilla in two batches.

6. Pop the tortillas into the oven until crisped, around 10 minutes. Remove from oven and keep warm.

7. Meanwhile, prepare salsa by mixing the remaining ingredients in a medium bowl. Stir to mix well.

To enjoy, dip crisped tortillas into bowl of salsa and eat or, you can spread the fruity salsa all over one tortilla chip and enjoy.

Nutrition: Calories 213 Fat 11g Carbs 25g Protein 5g Fiber 7g

51.   Braised Kale

Preparation Time: 10minutes
Cooking Time: 15 minutes
Servings 3
Ingredients:

- 2 to 3 tbsp. water
- 1 tbsp. coconut oil
- ½ sliced red pepper
- 2 stalk celery (sliced to ¼-inch thick)
- 5 cups of chopped kale

Instructions:

Heat a pan over medium heat.

Add coconut oil and sauté the celery for at least five minutes.

Add the kale and red pepper.

Add a tablespoon of water.

Let the vegetables wilt for a few minutes. Add a tablespoon of water if the kale starts to stick to the pan.

Serve warm.

Nutrition: Calories 61 Fat 5g Carbs 3g Protein 1g Fiber 1g

52.   Stir Fried Brussels sprouts and Carrots

Preparation Time: 10 minutes
Cooking time: 15 minutes
Servings: 6
Ingredients:

- 1 tbsp. cider vinegar
- 1/3 cup water
- 1 lb. Brussels sprouts, halved lengthwise
- 1 lb. carrots cut diagonally into ½-inch thick lengths
- 3 tbsp. olive oil, divided
- 2 tbsp. chopped shallot
- ½ tsp. pepper
- ¾ tsp. salt

Instructions:

1. On medium-high fire, place a nonstick medium fry pan and heat 2 tbsp. oil.
2. Ass shallots and cook until softened, around one to two minutes while occasionally stirring.
3. Add pepper salt, Brussels sprouts, and carrots. Stir fry until vegetables start to brown on the edges, around 3 to 4 minutes.
4. Add water, cook, and cover.
5. After 5 to 8 minutes, or when veggies are already soft, add remaining butter.
6. If needed, season with more pepper and salt to taste.
7. Turn off fire, transfer to a platter, serve and enjoy.

Nutrition: Calories 98 Fat 4g Carbs 14g Protein 3g Fiber 5g

53.   Curried Veggies and Poached Eggs

Preparation Time: 10 minutes
Cooking Time: 50 minutes
Servings: 4
Ingredients:

- 4 large eggs
- ½ tsp. white vinegar
- 1/8 tsp. crushed red pepper – optional
- 1 cup water
- 1 14-oz can chickpeas, drained
- 2 medium zucchinis, diced
- ½ lb. sliced button mushrooms
- 1 tbsp. yellow curry powder
- 2 cloves garlic, minced
- 1 large onion, chopped
- 2 tsp. extra virgin olive oil

Instructions:

1. On medium high fire, place a large saucepan and heat oil.

2. Sauté onions until tender around four to five minutes.

3. Add garlic and salt for another half minute.

4. Add curry powder, stir and cook until fragrant around one to two minutes.

5. Add mushrooms, mix, cover and cook for 5 to 8 minutes or until mushrooms are tender and have released their liquid.

6. Add red pepper if using, water, chickpeas and zucchini. Mix well to combine and bring to a boil.

7. Once boiling, reduce fire to a simmer, cover, and cook until zucchini is tender around 15 to 20 minutes of simmering.

8. Meanwhile, in a small pot filled with 3-inches deep of water, bring to a boil on a high fire.

9. Once boiling, reduce fire to a simmer and add vinegar.

10. Slowly add one egg, slipping it gently into the water. Allow to simmer until egg is cooked, around 3 to 5 minutes.

11. Remove egg with a slotted spoon and transfer to a plate, one plate one egg.

12. Repeat the process with remaining eggs.

13. Once the veggies are done cooking, divide evenly into 4 servings and place one serving per plate of egg.

14. Serve and enjoy.

Nutrition: Calories 254 Fat 9g Carbs 30g Protein 16g Fiber 9g

54. Braised Leeks, Cauliflower and Artichoke Hearts

Preparation Time: 10 minutes
Cooking Time: 10 minutes
Servings 4
Ingredients:

- 2 tbsp. coconut oil
- 2 garlic cloves, chopped
- 1 ½ cup artichoke hearts
- 1 ½ cups chopped leeks
- 1 ½ cups cauliflower flowerets

Instructions:

1. Heat oil in a skillet over medium-high heat.
2. Add the garlic and sauté for one minute. Add the vegetables and constantly stir until the vegetables are cooked.
3. Serve with roasted chicken, fish or pork.

Nutrition: Calories 111 Fat 7g Carbs 12g Protein 3g Fiber 4g

55. Celery Root Hash Browns

Preparation Time: 10 minutes
Cooking Time: 10 minutes
Servings 4
Ingredients:

- 4 tbsp. coconut oil
- ½ tsp. sea salt
- 2 to 3 medium celery roots

Instructions:

1. Scrub the celery root clean and peel it using a vegetable peeler.
2. Grate the celery root in a food processor or a manual grater.
3. In a skillet, add oil and heat it over medium heat.
4. Place the grated celery root on the skillet and sprinkle with salt.
5. Let it cook for 10 minutes on each side or until the grated celery turns brown.
6. Serve warm.

Nutrition: Calories 160 Fat 14g Carbs 10g Protein 1.5g Fiber 3g

56. Magic Green Falafels

Ingredients:

- One large onion, chopped
- 1 tsp. sea salt
- 2/3 cup fresh basil
- 1/2 cup fresh dill
- 2 cups dry garbanzo beans (chickpeas)
- 1/4 tsp. oregano
- 1/3 cup red bell pepper, chopped
- Grapeseed or avocado oil for frying
- 1/2 cup garbanzo bean flour

Instructions:

1. To make your Magic Green Falafels, start with cooking the chickpeas until they are soft. Drain the beans and rinse.
2. Place the chickpeas and all the other ingredients in a food processor: onion, red bell pepper, fresh herbs, sea salt, oregano, and flour.
3. Pulse until all the ingredients are thinly chopped and form a coarse meal. Scrape the sides down and pump again until the texture looks like a fine meal. Taste the seasonings and adjust if necessary.
4. Move the mixture into a large saucepan. Shape small balls or thick disks using your hands, and put them on a put lined with parchment paper—Chilla total of 1 hour in the refrigerator.
5. Fill a large skillet with oil; you want an approximate depth of 1 inch. Heat for about 5~7 minutes, over medium heat—Fry the Magic Green Falafels for 2~3 minutes per side, when the oil is hot.

57. Zucchini Pasta with Avocado Sauce

Preparations Time: 10 minutes

Cooking Time: 10 minutes

Servings: 1

Ingredients:

- A squeeze of lemon juice
- Salt and pepper to taste
- 1 tbsp. coconut milk
- ½ ripe avocado
- 1 medium zucchini cut into noodles
- 2 tbsp. olive oil

Instructions:

1. Heat the oil in a skillet over medium heat and add the zucchini noodles. Sauté for three minutes or until the noodles have softened.

2. While the zucchini is cooking, mash the avocado together with the coconut milk, lemon juice, and salt and pepper.
3. Add the sauce to the zucchini noodles and sauté. Serve warm.

Nutrition: Calories 471 Fat 43g Carbs 23g Protein 6g Fiber 9g

---

58.   Zucchini Garlic Fries

Preparation Time: 10 minutes
Cooking Time: 20 minutes
Servings: 6
Ingredients:

- ¼ teaspoon garlic powder
- ½ cup almond flour
- 2 large egg whites, beaten
- 3 medium zucchinis, sliced into fry sticks
- Salt and pepper to taste

Instructions:

1. Preheat oven to 400oF.
2. Mix all ingredients until the zucchini fries are well coated.
3. Place fries on cookie sheet and spread evenly.
4. Put in oven and cook for 20 minutes.
5. Halfway through cooking time, stir fries.

Nutrition: Calories 11 Fat 0.1g, Carbs 1g Protein 1.5 g Fiber 0.5g

---

59.   Avocado Coconut Pie

Preparation Time: 30 Minutes
Cooking Time: 50 Minutes
Servings: 4
Ingredients:
For the piecrust:

- 1 tbsp. flax seed powder + 3 tbsp. water
- 4 tbsp. coconut flour
- 4 tbsp. chia seeds
- ¾ cup almond flour

- 1 tbsp. psyllium husk powder
- 1 tsp. baking powder
- 1 pinch salt
- 3 tbsp. coconut oil
- 4 tbsp. water

For the filling:

- 2 ripe avocados
- 1 cup vegan mayonnaise
- 3 tbsp. flax seed powder + 9 tbsp. water
- 2 tbsp. fresh parsley, finely chopped

- 1 jalapeno, finely chopped
- ½ tsp. onion powder
- ¼ tsp. salt
- ½ cup cashew cream
- 1¼ cups shredded tofu cheese

Instructions:

1. In 2 separate bowls, mix the different portions of flax seed powder with the respective quantity of water. Allow absorbing for 5 minutes.
2. Preheat the oven to 350 F.
3. In a food processor, add the coconut flour, chia seeds, almond flour, psyllium husk powder, baking powder, salt, coconut oil, water, and the smaller portion of the flax egg. Blend the ingredients until the resulting dough forms into a ball.
4. Line a spring form pan with about 12-inch diameter of parchment paper and spread the dough in the pan.
5. Meanwhile, cut the avocado into halves lengthwise, remove the pit, and chop the pulp. Put in a bowl and add the mayonnaise, remaining flax egg, parsley, jalapeno, onion powder, salt, cashew cream, and tofu cheese. Combine well.
6. Remove the piecrust when ready and fill with the creamy mixture. Level the filling with a spatula and continue baking for 35 minutes or until lightly golden brown.
7. When ready, take out. Cool before slicing and serving with a baby spinach salad.

Nutrition: Calories: 680 Cal Fat: 71.8 g Carbs: 10 g Fiber: 7 g Protein: 3 g

CHAPTER 45

Smoothies and Beverages

SMOOTHIE 10~DAYS DETOX~PLANS

Days	Breakfast	Soup, Salad, & Sides	Smoothie
1	Omelet with Chickpea Flour	Coconut Watercress Soup	Energizing Ginger Detox Tonic
2	Tasty Oatmeal and Carrot Cake	Avocado Mint Soup	Fragrant Spiced Coffee
3	Onion & Mushroom Tart with a Nice Brown Rice Crust	Creamy Squash Soup	Tangy Spiced Cranberry Drink
4	Perfect Breakfast Shake	Cucumber Edamame Salad	Warm Pomegranate Punch
5	Beet Gazpacho	Best Broccoli Salad	Rich Truffle Hot Chocolate
6	Vegetable Rice	Rainbow Orzo Salad	Ultimate Mulled Wine
7	Courgette Risotto	Broccoli Pasta Salad	Pleasant Lemonade
8	Orange Dream Creamsicle	Tamari Toasted Almonds	Cantaloupe Smoothie Bowl
9	Strawberry Limeade	Nourishing Whole-Grain Porridge	Berry & Cauliflower Smoothie
10	Peanut Butter and Jelly Smoothie	Pungent Mushroom Barley Risotto	Green Mango Smoothie

60.   Fruity Smoothie

Preparation Time: 10 Minutes
Cooking time: 0 minute
Servings: 1
Ingredients:

- ¾ cup soy yogurt
- ½ cup pineapple juice
- 1 cup pineapple chunks
- 1 cup raspberries, sliced
- 1 cup blueberries, sliced

Instructions:

1. Process the ingredients in a blender.
2. Chill before serving.

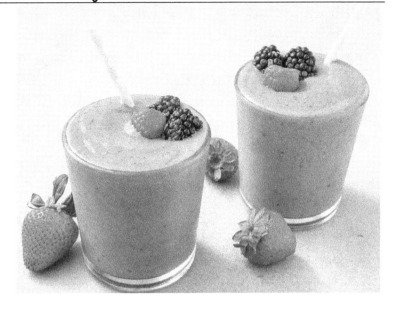

Nutrition: Calories 279, Total Fat 2 g, Saturated Fat 0 g   Cholesterol 4 mg, Sodium 149 mg, Total Carbohydrate 56 g   Dietary Fiber 7 g, Protein 12 g

61.   Energizing Ginger Detox Tonic

Preparation Time: 15 minutes
Cooking Time: 10 minutes
Servings: 2
Ingredients:

- 1/2 teaspoon of grated ginger, fresh
- 1 small lemon slice
- 1/8 teaspoon of cayenne pepper
- 1/8 teaspoon of ground turmeric
- 1/8 teaspoon of ground cinnamon
- 1 teaspoon of maple syrup
- 1 teaspoon of apple cider vinegar
- 2 cups of boiling water

Instructions:

1. Pour the boiling water into a small saucepan, add and stir the ginger, then let it rest for 8 to 10 minutes, before covering the pan.
2. Pass the mixture through a strainer and into the liquid, add the cayenne pepper, turmeric, cinnamon and stir properly.
3. Add the maple syrup, vinegar, and lemon slice.
4. Add and stir an infused lemon and serve immediately.

Nutrition: Calories:80 Cal, Carbohydrates:0g, Protein:0g, Fats:0g, Fiber:0g

---

62.　　Warm Spiced Lemon Drink

Preparation Time: 2 hours and 10 minutes
Cooking Time: 2 hours
Servings: 12
Ingredients:

- 1 cinnamon stick, about 3 inches long
- 1/2 teaspoon of whole cloves
- 2 cups of coconut sugar
- 4 fluid of ounce pineapple juice
- 1/2 cup and 2 tablespoons of lemon juice
- 12 fluid ounce of orange juice
- 2 1/2 quarts of water

Instructions:

1. Pour water into a 6-quarts slow cooker and stir the sugar and lemon juice properly.
2. Wrap the cinnamon, the whole cloves in cheesecloth and tie its corners with string.
3. Immerse this cheesecloth bag in the liquid present in the slow cooker and cover it with the lid.
4. Then plug in the slow cooker and let it cook on high heat setting for 2 hours or until it is heated thoroughly.
5. When done, discard the cheesecloth bag and serve the drink hot or cold.

Nutrition: Calories:15 Cal, Carbohydrates:3.2g, Protein:0.1g, Fats:0g, Fiber:0g.

63.   Soothing Ginger Tea Drink

Preparation Time: 2 hours and 15 minutes
Cooking Time: 2 hours and 10 minutes
Servings: 8
Ingredients:

- 1 tablespoon of minced ginger root
- 2 tablespoons of honey
- 15 green tea bags
- 32 fluid ounce of white grape juice
- 2 quarts of boiling water

Instructions:

1. Pour water into a 4-quarts slow cooker, immerse tea bags, cover the cooker and let stand for 10 minutes.
2. After 10 minutes, remove and discard tea bags and stir in remaining ingredients.
3. Return cover to slow cooker, then plug in and let cook at high heat setting for 2 hours or until heated through.
4. When done, strain the liquid and serve hot or cold.

Nutrition: Calories:45 Cal, Carbohydrates:12g, Protein:0g, Fats:0g, Fiber:0g

64.   Nice Spiced Cherry Cider

Preparation Time: 4 hours and 5 minutes
Cooking Time: 4 hours
Servings: 16
Ingredients:

- 2 cinnamon sticks
- 6-ounce of cherry gelatin
- 4 quarts of apple cider

Instructions:

1. Using a 6-quarts slow cooker, pour the apple cider and add the cinnamon stick.
2. Stir, then cover the slow cooker with its lid. Plug in the cooker and let it cook for 3 hours at the high heat setting or until it is heated thoroughly.

3. Then add and stir the gelatin properly, then continue cooking for another hour.

4. When done, remove the cinnamon sticks and serve the drink hot or cold.

Nutrition: Calories:100 Cal, Carbohydrates:0g, Protein:0g, Fats:0g, Fiber:0g.

65. Fragrant Spiced Coffee

Preparation Time: 3 hours and 10 minutes
Cooking Time: 3 hours
Servings: 8
Ingredients:

1/2 teaspoons of whole cloves

1/3 cup of honey

2-ounce of chocolate syrup

1/2 teaspoon of anise extract

8 cups of brewed coffee

Instructions:

1. Pour the coffee in a 4-quarts slow cooker and pour in the remaining ingredients except for cinnamon and stir properly.

2. Wrap the whole cloves in cheesecloth and tie its corners with strings.

3. Immerse this cheesecloth bag in the liquid present in the slow cooker and cover it with the lid.

4. Then plug in the slow cooker and let it cook on the low heat setting for 3 hours or until heated thoroughly.

5. When done, discard the cheesecloth bag and serve.

Nutrition: Calories:150 Cal, Carbohydrates:35g, Protein:3g, Fats:0g, Fiber:0g

66. Tangy Spiced Cranberry Drink

Preparation Time: 3 hours and 10 minutes
Cooking Time: 3 hours
Servings: 14
Ingredients:

- 1 1/2 cups of coconut sugar
- 12 whole cloves
- 2 fluid ounce of lemon juice
- 6 fluid ounce of orange juice
- 32 fluid ounces of cranberry juice
- 8 cups of hot water
- 1/2 cup of Red-Hot candies

Instructions:

1. Pour the water into a 6-quarts slow cooker along with the cranberry juice, orange juice, and the lemon juice.
2. Stir the sugar properly.
3. Wrap the whole cloves in a cheese cloth, tie its corners with strings, and immerse it in the liquid present inside the slow cooker.
4. Add the red-hot candies to the slow cooker and cover it with the lid.
5. Then plug in the slow cooker and let it cook on the low heat setting for 3 hours or until it is heated thoroughly.
6. When done, discard the cheesecloth bag and serve.

Nutrition: Calories:89 Cal, Carbohydrates:27g, Protein:0g, Fats:0g, Fiber:1g.

67. Warm Pomegranate Punch

Preparation Time: 3 hours and 15 minutes
Cooking time: 3 hours
Servings: 10
Ingredients:

- 3 cinnamon sticks, each about 3 inches long
- 12 whole cloves
- 1/2 cup of coconut sugar
- 1/3 cup of lemon juice
- 32 fluid ounce of pomegranate juice
- 32 fluid ounce of apple juice, unsweetened
- 16 fluid ounce of brewed tea

Instructions:

1. Using a 4-quart slow cooker, pour the lemon juice, pomegranate, juice apple juice, tea, and then sugar.
2. Wrap the whole cloves and cinnamon stick in a cheese cloth, tie its corners with a string, and immerse it in the liquid present in the slow cooker.
3. Then cover it with the lid, plug in the slow cooker and let it cook at the low heat setting for 3 hours or until it is heated thoroughly.
4. When done, discard the cheesecloth bag and serve it hot or cold.

Nutrition: Calories:253 Cal, Carbohydrates:58g, Protein:7g, Fats:2g, Fiber:3g.

---

68.   Rich Truffle Hot Chocolate

Preparation Time: 2 hours and 10 minutes
Cooking time: 2 hours
Servings: 4
Ingredients:

- 1/3 cup of cocoa powder, unsweetened
- 1/3 cup of coconut sugar
- 1/8 teaspoon of salt
- 1/8 teaspoon of ground cinnamon
- 1 teaspoon of vanilla extract, unsweetened
- 32 fluid ounce of coconut milk

Instructions:

1. Using a 2 quarts slow cooker, add all the ingredients and stir properly.
2. Cover it with the lid, then plug in the slow cooker and cook it for 2 hours on the high heat setting or until it is heated thoroughly.
3. When done, serve right away.

Nutrition: Calories:67 Cal, Carbohydrates:13g, Protein:2g, Fats:2g, Fiber:2.3g.

69.   Ultimate Mulled Wine

Preparation Time: 35 minutes
Cooking time: 30 minutes
Servings: 6
Ingredients:

- 1 cup of cranberries, fresh
- 2 oranges, juiced
- 1 tablespoon of whole cloves
- 1 tablespoon of star anise
- 1/3 cup of honey
- 8 fluid ounce of apple cider
- 8 fluid ounce of cranberry juice
- 24 fluid ounce of red wine

Instructions:

1. Using a 4 quarts slow cooker, add all the ingredients and stir properly.
2. Cover it with the lid, then plug in the slow cooker and cook it for 30 minutes on thee high heat setting or until it gets warm thoroughly.
3. When done, strain the wine and serve right away.

Nutrition: Calories:202 Cal, Carbohydrates:25g, Protein:0g, Fats:0g, Fiber:0g

70.   Coconut & Strawberry Smoothie

Preparation Time: 10 Minutes
Cooking Time: 0 minutes
Serves: 1
Ingredients:

- 1 Cup Strawberries, Frozen & Thawed Slightly
- 1 Ripe Banana, Sliced & Frozen
- ½ Cup Coconut Milk, Light
- ½ Cup Vegan Yogurt
- 1 Tablespoon Chia Seeds
- 1 Teaspoon Lime juice, Fresh
- 4 Ice Cubes

Instructions:

1. Blend all ingredients together until smooth, and serve immediately.

Nutrition: Calories: 278 Protein: 14 Grams Fat: 2 Grams Carbs: 57 Grams

71.   Pleasant Lemonade

Preparation Time: 3 hours and 15 minutes
Cooking time: 3 hours
Servings: 10 servings
Ingredients:

- Cinnamon sticks for serving
- 2 cups of coconut sugar
- 1/4 cup of honey
- 3 cups of lemon juice. fresh
- 32 fluid ounce of water

Instructions:

1. Using a 4-quarts slow cooker, place all the ingredients except for the cinnamon sticks and stir properly.
2. Cover it with the lid, then plug in the slow cooker and cook it on the low heat setting or until it is heated thoroughly.
3. When done, stir properly and serve with the cinnamon sticks.

Nutrition: Calories:146 Cal, Carbohydrates:34g, Protein:0g, Fats:0g, Fiber:0g.

72.   Pumpkin Chia Smoothie

Preparation Time: 5 Minutes
Cooking Time: 0 minutes
Serves: 1
Ingredients:

- 3 Tablespoons Pumpkin Puree
- 1 Tablespoon MCT Oil
- ¾ Cup Coconut Milk, Full Fat
- ½ Avocado, Fresh
- 1 Teaspoon Vanilla, Pure
- ½ Teaspoon Pumpkin Pie Spice

Instructions:

Combine all ingredients together until blended.

Nutrition: Calories: 726 Protein: 5.5 Grams Fat: 69.8 Grams Carbs: 15 Grams

73.   Pineapple, Banana & Spinach Smoothie

Preparation Time: 10 Minutes
Cooking time: 0 minute
Servings: 1
Ingredients:

- ½ cup almond milk
- ¼ cup soy yogurt
- 1 cup spinach
- 1 cup banana
- 1 cup pineapple chunks
- 1 tbsp. chia seeds

Instructions:

1. Add all the ingredients in a blender.
2. Blend until smooth.
3. Chill in the refrigerator before serving.

Nutrition: Calories 297, Total Fat 6 g, Saturated Fat 1 g, Cholesterol 4 mg   Sodium 145 mg, Total Carbohydrate 54 g, Dietary Fiber 10 g   Protein 13 g, Total Sugars 29g, Potassium 1038 mg

74.   Kale & Avocado Smoothie

Preparation Time: 10 Minutes
Cooking time: 0 minute
Servings: 1
Ingredients:

- 1 ripe banana
- 1 cup kale
- 1 cup almond milk
- ¼ avocado
- 1 tbsp. chia seeds
- 2 tsp. honey
- 1 cup ice cubes

Instructions:

1. Blend all the ingredients until smooth.

Nutrition: Calories 343 Total Fat 14 g   Saturated Fat 2 g   Cholesterol 0 mg   Sodium 199 mg   Total Carbohydrate 55 g   Dietary Fiber 12 g   Protein 6 g   Total Sugars 29 g   Potassium 1051 mg

75.   Cantaloupe Smoothie Bowl

Preparation Time: 5 Minutes
Cooking Time: 0 minutes
Serves: 2
Ingredients:

- ¾ Cup carrot Juice
- 4 Cps Cantaloupe, Frozen & Cubed
- Mellon Balls or Berries to Serve
- Pinch Sea Salt

Instructions:

2. Blend everything together until smooth.

Nutrition: Calories: 135 Protein: 3 Grams Fat: 1 Gram Carbs: 32 Grams

76.   Chia Seed Smoothie

Preparation Time: 5 Minutes
Cooking Time: 0 minutes
Serves: 3
Ingredients:

- ¼ Teaspoon Cinnamon
- 1 Tablespoon Ginger, Fresh & Grated
- Pinch Cardamom
- 1 Tablespoon Chia Seeds
- 2 Medjool Dates, Pitted
- 1 Cup Alfalfa Sprouts
- 1 Cup Water
- 1 Banana
- ½ Cup Coconut Milk, Unsweetened

Instructions:

Blend everything together until smooth.

Nutrition: Calories: 477 Protein: 8 Grams Fat: 29 Grams Carbs: 57 Grams

77.   Berry & Cauliflower Smoothie

Preparation Time: 10 Minutes
Cooking Time: 0 minutes
Serves: 2
Ingredients:
1 Cup Riced Cauliflower, Frozen
1 Cup Banana, Sliced & Frozen
½ Cup Mixed Berries, Frozen
2 Cups Almond Milk, Unsweetened
2 Teaspoons Maple syrup, Pure & Optional
Instructions:
Blend until mixed well.

Nutrition: Calories: 149 Protein: 3 Grams Fat: 3 Grams Carbs: 29 Grams

78.   Green Mango Smoothie

Preparation Time: 5 Minutes
Cooking Time: 0 minutes
Serves: 1
Ingredients:
2 Cups Spinach
1-2 Cups Coconut Water
2 Mangos, Ripe, Peeled & Diced
Instructions:
Blend everything together until smooth.

Nutrition: Calories: 417 Protein: 7.2 Grams Fat: 2.8 Grams Carbs: 102.8 Grams

79.   Mango Smoothie

Preparation Time: 5 Minutes
Cooking Time: 0 minutes
Serves: 3
Ingredients:

- 1 Carrot, Peeled & Chopped
- 1 Cup Strawberries
- 1 Cup Water
- 1 Cup Peaches, Chopped
- 1 Banana, Frozen & sliced
- 1 Cup Mango, Chopped

Instructions:

Blend everything together until smooth.

Nutrition: Calories: 376 Protein: 5 Grams Fat: 2 Grams Carbs: 95 Grams

CHAPTER 46

Desserts and Snacks

80. Chickpeas Salad

Preparation Time: 5 minutes
Cooking time: 0 minutes
Servings: 4
Ingredients:

- 2 cups canned chickpeas, drained and rinsed
- 1 tablespoon capers, chopped
- 2 tablespoons lime juice
- 2 tablespoons olive oil
- 4 spring onions, chopped
- 1 teaspoon chili powder
- 1 teaspoon cumin, ground
- 1 tablespoon parsley, chopped
- A pinch of salt and black pepper

Instructions:

In a bowl, combine the chickpeas and capers and the other ingredients, toss and serve as a side salad.

Nutrition: Calories: 212 Cal Fat: 4 g Fiber: 4 g Carbs: 12 g Protein: 6 g

81.   Quinoa and Beans

Preparation Time: 10 minutes
Cooking time: 30 minutes
Servings: 4
Ingredients:

- 1 tablespoon olive oil
- 1 yellow onion, chopped
- 1 cup quinoa
- ½ cup canned black beans, drained and rinsed
- 2 cups chicken stock
- 2 garlic cloves, minced
- Salt and black pepper to the taste
- 1 tablespoon cilantro, chopped

Instructions:

1. Heat up a pan with the olive oil over medium heat, add the onion and the garlic and sauté for 5 minutes.

2. Add the quinoa and the other ingredients, toss,and cook over medium heat for 25 minutes.

3. Divide everything between plates and serve.

Nutrition: Calories: 212 Cal Fat: 1 g Fiber: 2 g Carbs: 2 g Protein: 1 g

82.   Barley and Kale

Preparation Time: 5 minutes
Cooking Time: 0 minutes
Servings: 4
Ingredients:

- 2 cups barley, cooked
- 1 cup baby kale
- 2 tablespoons almonds, chopped
- 2 tablespoons balsamic vinegar
- 1 tablespoon olive oil
- 1 tablespoon cilantro, chopped

Instructions:

In a bowl, mix the barley with the kale, the almonds and the other ingredients, toss and serve as a side dish.

Nutrition: Calories: 175 Cal Fat: 3 g Fiber: 3 g Carbs: 5 g Protein: 6 g

83.   Fancy Coconut Date Bars for a Lovely Evening

Preparation Time: 10 Minutes
Cooking Time: 30 Minutes
Servings: 4
Ingredients:

- 1/3 cup of slivered almonds
- ½ a cup coconut, flaked
- 10 dates, pitted
- ¼ cup of cashews
- 1 teaspoon of coconut oil

Instructions:

1. Take a food processor and ad the almonds, blend them
2. Add dates and pulse until mixed well
3. Add coconut oil and cashews until the mix is thick and sticks together
4. Transfer the mixture to a wax paper and form nice squares
5. Fold up the sides of the waxed-on top
6. serve and Enjoy!

Nutrition: Calories: 154 Cal Fats: 0 g Carbs: 39 g Protein: 0.1 g

84.   Vegan Coconut Whipped Cream

Preparation Time: 8 Hours 10 Minutes
Cooking Time: 0
Servings: 6
Ingredients

- 1 can of unsweetened coconut milk
- 2 tablespoons of white sugar
- 1 teaspoon of pure vanilla extract

Instructions:

1. Place the can of coconut in your fridge and allow it to chill for 8 hours
2. Make sure to chill a metal bowl and beats in your fridge for about 1 hour prior to preparing the whip
3. Open up your coconut milk can and scoop out the coconut cream solids into your metal bowl
4. Keep the liquids for later use
5. Beat the cream using a mixer on medium speed
6. Set the speed on HIGH and beat for 7-8 minutes until stiff peaks form
7. Add sugar, vanilla extract to the coconut cream and beat for 1 minute more
8. Give it a taste and add more sugar if needed
Enjoy with cakes of muffins!

Nutrition: Calories: 11 Cal Fats: 0 g Carbs: 2.4 g Protein: 0 g

85. Tharp She' Salts Peanut Butter Cookies

Preparation Time: 15 Minutes
Cooking Time: 0
Servings: 9
Ingredients

- 1 cup of raw almonds
- ½ a cup of peanut butter (creamy and unsalted)
- 1 cup of pitted Mejdool dates
- 1 and a ¼ teaspoon of vanilla extract
- Sea salt as needed

Instructions:

1. Take a food processor and add almonds, peanut butter, vanilla, dates and blend the whole mixture until a dough like texture comes (should take a few minutes)
2. Add some more peanut butter if you want a stickier dough
3. Form balls using the dough and press down using fork to create a crass cross pattern
4. Sprinkle salt generously
5. Serve instantly or allow it to chill for crunchiness

Nutrition: Calories: 350 Cal Fat: 17 g Carbs: 27 g Protein: 18 g

86. A Snowy "Frozen" Salad Bowl

Preparation Time: 75 Minutes
Cooking Time: 0
Servings: 3
Ingredients:

- ½ a cup of white sugar
- 2 cups of water
- 1 can of 20-ounce frozen orange juice concentrate (thawed)
- 1 can of 20-ounce frozen lemonade concentrated (thawed)
- 4 bananas, sliced
- 1 can have crushed pineapple (with juice)
- 1 pack of strawberries (thawed)

Instructions:

1. Prepare water and sugar
2. Dissolve the sugar and add orange juice, bananas, lemonade, crushed pineapples (alongside the juice), and strawberries and give it a nice mix
3. Pour the mixture into a 9x13 inch glass pan and allow it to chill
4. Once ready to serve, let it sit for about 5 minutes at room temp and cut them out

Nutrition: Calories: 350 Cal Fats: 0.5 g Carbs: 89 g Protein: 2.5 g

---

87. Warm Mushroom and Orange Pepper Salad

Preparation Time: 10 Minutes
Cooking Time: 8 Minutes
Servings: 4
Ingredients:

- 2 tbsp. avocado oil
- 1 cup mixed mushrooms, chopped
- 2 orange bell peppers, deseeded and finely sliced
- 1 garlic clove, minced
- 2 tbsp. tamarind sauce
- 1 tsp. maple (sugar-free) syrup
- ½ tsp. hot sauce
- ½ tsp. fresh ginger paste
- Sesame seeds to garnish

Instructions:

1. Over medium fire, heat half of avocado oil in a large skillet, sauté mushroom and bell peppers until slightly softened, 5 minutes.
2. In a small bowl, whisk garlic, tamarind sauce, maple syrup, hot sauce, and ginger paste. Add mixture to vegetables and stir-fry for 2 to 3 minutes.
3. Turn heat off and dish salad. Drizzle with remaining avocado oil and garnish with sesame seeds.
4. Serve with grilled tofu.

Nutrition: Calories: 289 Cal Fat: 26.71 g Carbs: 9 g Fiber: 3.8 g Protein: 4.23 g

88.   Broccoli, Kelp, and Feta Salad

Preparation Time: 15 Minutes
Cooking Time: 0
Servings: 4
Ingredients:

- 2 tbsp. olive oil
- 1 tbsp. white wine vinegar
- 2 tbsp. chia seeds
- 2 cups broccoli slaw
- 1 cup chopped kelp, thoroughly washed and steamed
- 1/3 cup chopped pecans
- 1/3 cup pumpkin seeds
- 1/3 cup blueberries
- 2/3 cup ricotta cheese

Instructions:

Whisk olive oil, white wine vinegar, chia seeds, salt, and black pepper. Set aside. Combine the broccoli slaw, kelp, pecans, pumpkin seeds, blueberries, and ricotta cheese.

Drizzle dressing on top, toss, and serve.

Nutrition: Calories 397 Fat 3.87g Carbs 8.4g Fiber 3.5g Protein 8.93g

89.   Roasted Asparagus with Feta Cheese Salad

Preparation Time: 10 minutes
Cooking Time: 20 minutes
Serving: 4
Ingredients:

- 1 lb. asparagus, trimmed and halved
- 2 tbsp. olive oil
- ½ tsp. dried basil
- ½ tsp. dried oregano
- ½ tsp. hemp seeds
- 1 tbsp. maple (sugar-free) syrup
- ½ cup arugula
- 4 tbsp. crumbled feta cheese
- 2 tbsp. hazelnuts
- 1 lemon, cut into wedges

Instructions:

1. Preheat oven to 350oF.
2. Pour asparagus on a baking tray, drizzle with olive oil, basil, oregano, salt, black pepper, and hemp seeds. Mix with your hands and roast in oven for 15 minutes.
3. Remove, drizzle with maple syrup, and continue cooking until slightly charred, 5 minutes.
4. Spread arugula in a salad bowl and top with asparagus. Scatter with feta cheese, hazelnuts, and serve with lemon wedges.

Nutrition: Calories: 146 Cal Fat: 12.87 g   Carbs: 5.07 g Fiber: 1.6 g Protein: 4.44 g

---

90.　　Fresh Veggie Salad

Preparation Time: 20 Minutes
Cooking Time: 0
Servings: 8
Ingredients:
For Dressing:

- 5 tablespoons olive oil
- 3 tablespoons fresh lemon juice
- 2 tablespoons fresh mint leaves, chopped finely
- 1 teaspoon Erythritol

For Salad:

- 2 cups cucumbers, peeled and sliced
- 2 cups tomatoes, sliced
- 1 cup black olives
- 6 cups lettuce
- 1 cup mozzarella cheese, cubed

Instructions:

1. For dressing: in a bowl, add all ingredients and beat until well combined.
2. Cover and refrigerate to chill for about 1 hour.
3. For the salad: add all ingredients and mix.
4. Discharge dressing over salad and toss to coat well.
5. Serve immediately.

Nutrition: Calories: 124 Cal Fat: 11.4 g Carbs: 5.4 g Protein: 2 g

91.   Strawberry Salad

Preparation Time: 15 Minutes
Cooking Time: 0
Servings: 4
Ingredients:

- 6 cups fresh baby greens
- 2 cups fresh strawberries, hulled and sliced
- 1 tablespoon fresh mint leaves
- ¼ cup olive oil
- 2 tablespoons fresh lemon juice
- ¼ teaspoon liquid stevia
- 1/8 teaspoon paprika
- 1/8 teaspoon garlic powder
- Salt, to taste

Instructions:

For the salad: add greens, strawberries, and mint and mix.
For dressing: in a bowl, add remaining ingredients and beat until well combined.
Discharge dressing over salad and toss to coat well.
Serve immediately.

Nutrition: Calories: 141 Cal Fat: 14.7 g Carbs: 1.8 g Protein: 2 g

92.   Cucumber and Green Onions Salad

Preparation Time: 5 minutes
Cooking Time: 0
Servings: 4
Ingredients:

- 2 tablespoons olive oil
- 2 cucumbers, sliced
- 4 spring onions, chopped
- ½ cup cilantro, chopped
- ½ cup lemon juice
- Salt and black pepper to the taste

Instructions:

In a salad bowl, combine the cucumbers with the spring onions and the other ingredients, toss and serve.

Nutrition: Calories: 163 Cal Fat: 1 g Fiber: 2 g Carbs: 7 g Protein: 9 g

93. Tex Mex Black Bean and Avocado Salad

Preparation Time: 15 Minutes
Cooking Time: 0
Servings: 2
Ingredients

- 14 oz. black beans, drained and rinsed
- 3 jars roasted red peppers, chopped
- 1 avocado, chopped
- ½ onion, chopped
- 1 red chili, chopped
- 1 lime, plus wedges to serve
- Olive oil
- 1 teaspoon cumin seeds
- 2 handfuls rocket
- 2 pitta breads, warmed

Instructions:

1. Combine beans, peppers, avocado, onion and chili in a large mixing bowl.
2. Add lime juice, cumin seeds and mix well.
3. Serve the rocket on two plates with warm pittas and divide the bean mixture.

Nutrition: Calories: 120 Cal   Fat: 3 g Fiber: 5 g Carbs: 3 g Protein: 5 g

94.   Sweet Potato Salad

Preparation: 10 Minutes
Cooking Time: 30 Minutes
Servings: 4
Ingredients:

- 2 sweet potatoes, peeled and cubed
- 1 tablespoon olive oil
- ½ teaspoon each of paprika, oregano and cayenne pepper
- 1 shallot, diced
- 2 spring onions, chopped
- 1 small bunch chives, chopped
- 3 tablespoons red wine vinegar
- 2 teaspoons olive oil
- 1 tablespoon pure maple syrup
- Salt and pepper

Instructions:

1. Prepare a baking sheet by lining it with parchment paper.
2. Place sweet potatoes in the baking sheet.
3. Drizzle some olive oil and spices, toss well and bake for 30 minutes.
4. In a separate bowl, mix shallots, scallions, chives, vinegar, olive oil and maple syrup.
5. Add baked sweet potatoes to the dressing.

Nutrition: Calories: 162 Cal   Fat: 8.0 g Fiber: 2.3 g Carbs: 6.3 g Protein: 8.1 g

95.   Lentil Fattoush Salad

Preparation Time: 10 Minutes
Cooking Time: 42 Minutes
Servings: 2
Ingredients:

- ⅓ cup dried green lentils
- 1 bag of whole wheat pita bread, cut into small pieces
- 2 teaspoons olive oil
- 2 teaspoons za'atar
- 4 cups loosely packed arugula
- 2 stalks celery, chopped
- 1 carrot stick, chopped
- ¼ small hothouse cucumber, chopped
- 1 small radish, thinly sliced
- ¼ cup dates, chopped
- 2 tablespoons toasted sunflower seeds
- For the maple Dijon vinaigrette:
- 2 tablespoons olive oil
- 2 tablespoons balsamic vinegar
- 1 tablespoon Dijon mustard
- 1 tablespoon maple syrup

Instructions:

1. Place a small pot over medium heat. Add lentils and 2/3 cup water.
2. Boil, lower the heat and bring it to a simmer for 35 minutes.
3. Preheat the oven to 425F. Line a baking sheet with parchment paper.
4. Mix pita pieces with olive oil and zaatar. Place on a baking sheet and bake for 7 minutes.
5. Mix arugula, lentils, veggies, dates, sunflower seeds and pita croutons.
6. Meanwhile in a separate bowl, mix the dressing ingredients and set aside.
7. Add the dressing and toss well before serving.

Nutrition: Calories: 154 Cal Fat: 8.4 g Fiber: 4.4 g Carbs: 4.3 g Protein: 7.1 g

96.   Lentil Salad with Spinach and Pomegranate

Preparation Time: 15 Minutes
Cooking Time: 0
Servings: 3
Ingredients
For the vegan lentil salad:

- 3 cups brown lentils, cooked
- 1 avocado, cut into slices
- 2-3 handfuls fresh spinach
- ½ cup walnuts, chopped
- 2 apples, chopped
- 1 pomegranate

For the tahini orange dressing:

- 3 tablespoons tahini
- 2 tablespoons olive oil
- 1 clove of garlic
- 6 tablespoons water
- 4 tablespoons orange juice
- 2 teaspoons orange zest
- Salt and pepper

Instructions:

1. Prepare lentils according to package instructions.
2. Place pomegranate in a shallow bowl filled with water, cut in half and take out seeds, remove fibers floating on the water.
3. Process all dressing ingredients in a food processor. Process until smooth and set aside.
4. Place salad ingredients in a large bowl and mix well.
5. Drizzle dressing over salad before serving.

Nutrition: Calories: 104 Cal Fat: 5 g Fiber: 4 g Carbs: 3.1 g Protein: 7.1 g

97.   Broccoli Salad Curry Dressing

Preparation Time: 30 Minutes
Cooking Time: 0
Servings: 6
Ingredients

- ½ cup plain, unsweetened vegan yogurt
- ¼ cup onion, chopped
- 2 heads broccoli florets, chopped
- 2 stalks celery, chopped
- ½ teaspoon curry powder
- ¼ teaspoon salt or to taste
- 2 tablespoons sunflower seeds

Instructions:

1. Mix yogurt, curry powder, and salt.
2. Toss broccoli florets, celery onion, and sunflower seeds.
3. Drizzle the dressing on top and put the salad in the fridge for 30 minutes.

Nutrition: Calories: 153 Cal Fat: 4 g Fiber: 3 g Carbs: 2 g Protein: 9.1 g

98.   Age Old Poached Pears

Preparation Time: 3 Minutes
Cooking Time: 17 Minutes
Servings: 4
Ingredients

- 3 semi ripe pears (preferably Barlett pears)
- 3 and a ½ cups of water
- 3 cups of granulated sugar
- Rind of 1 lemon
- Juice of 1 lemon
- 1 teaspoon of vanilla extract
- 2 cinnamon sticks
- 2 pieces of whole cloves
- 1 whole star anise

Instructions:

1. Peel your pears and keep them on the side
2. Take a pot and add vanilla extract, water, lemon juice, sugar, lemon rind, star anise, cinnamon sticks, and cloves
3. Place it over medium heat and keep Cook until the sugar dissolves
4. Add your peas and lower down the heat to low
5. Allow it to simmer for 15-20 minutes
6. Once the pears are soft, transfer to a Tupperware with Cook liquid
7. Allow it to cool
Serve and enjoy!

Nutrition: Calories: 740 Cal Fat: 4 g Carbs: 180 g Protein: 4 g

99.   A Pineapple "Sherbet" If You Please

Preparation Time: 20 Minutes
Cooking Time: 0
Servings: 4
Ingredients

- 1 can of 8-ounce pineapple chunks
- 1/3 cup of orange marmalade
- ¼ teaspoon of ground ginger
- ¼ teaspoon of vanilla extract
- 1 can of 11-ounce orange sections
- 2 cups of pineapple, lemon or lime sherbet

Instructions:

1. Take a medium sized bowl and add pineapple juice, ginger, vanilla and marmalade to the bowl
3. Add pineapple chunks, drained mandarin oranges as well
4. Toss well and coat everything
5. Free them for 15 minutes and allow them to chill
6. Spoon the sherbet into 4 chilled stemmed sherbet dishes
7. Top each of them with fruit mixture
Enjoy!

Nutrition: Calories: 267 Cal Fat: 1 g Carbs: 65 g Protein: 2 g

100. Very Rough and Tough Fried Apple

Preparation Time: 10 Minutes
Cooking Time: 10 Minute
Servings: 4
Ingredients

½ a cup of vegan butter
½ a cup of white sugar
2 tablespoon of ground cinnamon

4 Granny Smith Apples, peeled, sliced and cored

Instructions:

1. Take a large-sized skillet and place it over medium heat
2. Add the vegan butter and allow it to melt
3. Stir in cinnamon and sugar into the melted butter
4. Add the cut-up apples and cook them nicely for about 5-8 minutes until they break down

Enjoy!

Nutrition: Calories: 369 Cal Fat: 23 g Carbs: 44 g Protein: 1 g

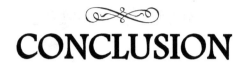

CONCLUSION

Congratulations! Now you have learned 100 simple, Doctor Sebi alkaline diet recipes. That means you can surprise yourself, your family, and your friends with new, delicious dishes, snacks, salads, desserts, or smoothies. Not only will you be eating tasty meals, you will also be helping yourself and your family to feel better and improve overall health just by eating approved Doctor Sebi food.

How great is that?

Now there is just one thing for you to do: Take action!

I know, you have most likely been in this position before. Maybe you have already tried other diets in the past, but you just can't find a suitable

Nutritional plan for you.

This time will be different. I promise!

Take care of yourself and live a long, healthy life!

CPSIA information can be obtained
at www.ICGtesting.com
Printed in the USA
LVHW101110291220
675196LV00013B/722

9 781801 324229